Treating and Beating Heart Disease: A Consumer's Guide to Cardiac Medicines

Barbara H. Roberts, MD, FACC
Director, The Women's Cardiac Center
The Miriam Hospital
Providence, RI

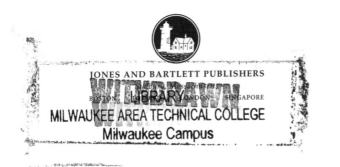

JONES AND BARTLETT PUBLISHERS
BOSTON   LONDON   SINGAPORE

World Headquarters

Jones and Bartlett Publishers	Jones and Bartlett Publishers	Jones and Bartlett Publishers
40 Tall Pine Drive	Canada	International
Sudbury, MA 01776	6339 Ormindale Way	Barb House, Barb Mews
978-443-5000	Mississauga, Ontario L5V 1J2	London W6 7PA
info@jbpub.com	Canada	UK
www.jbpub.com		

Jones and Bartlett's books and products are available through most bookstores and online book-sellers. To contact Jones and Bartlett Publishers directly, call 800-832-0034, fax 978-443-8000, or visit our website www.jbpub.com.

Substantial discounts on bulk quantities of Jones and Bartlett's publications are available to corporations, professional associations, and other qualified organizations. For details and specific discount information, contact the special sales department at Jones and Bartlett via the above contact information or send an email to specialsales@jbpub.com.

The authors, editor, and publisher have made every effort to provide accurate information. However, they are not responsible for errors, omissions, or for any outcomes related to the use of the contents of this book and take no responsibility for the use of the products and procedures described. Treatments and side effects described in this book may not be applicable to all people; likewise, some people may require a dose or experience a side effect that is not described herein. Drugs and medical devices are discussed that may have limited availability controlled by the Food and Drug Administration (FDA) for use only in a research study or clinical trial. Research, clinical practice, and government regulations often change the accepted standard in this field. When consideration is being given to use of any drug in the clinical setting, the health care provider or reader is responsible for determining FDA status of the drug, reading the package insert, and reviewing prescribing information for the most up-to-date recommendations on dose, precautions, and contraindications, and determining the appropriate usage for the product. This is especially important in the case of drugs that are new or seldom used.

CIP Data not available at time of printing.

Production Credits
Executive Editor: Christopher Davis
Acquisitions Editor: Janice Hackenberg
Production Director: Amy Rose
Associate Production Editor: Rachel Rossi
Editorial Assistant: Jessica Acox
Associate Marketing Manager: Ilana Goddess
Manufacturing Buyer: Therese Connell
Composition: Publishers' Design and Production Services, Inc.
Cover Design: Kate Ternullo
Cover Image: © DJAPEMAN/Shutterstock, Inc.
Printing and Binding: Malloy, Inc.
Cover Printing: Malloy, Inc.

Printed in the United States of America
12 11 10 09 08   10 9 8 7 6 5 4 3 2 1

Dedication

In memory of my father:
Alan Raymond Hudson, 1920–2006

Contents

Acknowledgments

I would like to thank Janice Hackenberg, Jessica Acox, Christopher Davis, and Rachel Rossi of Jones and Bartlett for making this book possible and readable. My staff at The Women's Cardiac Center at The Miriam Hospital, nurse practitioners Patricia Shea Leary and Joan Brennan, and secretary Becky Aucoin are joys to work with. I cannot thank them enough.

Dr. Kathleen Hittner, president and CEO, and Sandra Coletta, chief operating officer, both of The Miriam Hospital have been unfailingly supportive of the work we do at The Women's Cardiac Center. My gratitude goes to my colleagues in the division of cardiology who free up my time and energy for writing by taking night and weekend call, including Drs. Kenneth Korr, Paul Gordon, Peter Tilkemeier, Immad Sadiq, John Elion, Tom Crain, Douglas Burtt, Harry Schwartz, and Gary Katzman.

Sally Lapides and Joe Caramadre were there for me when I needed them. I will forever be grateful for their support and friendship.

As always, the love and support of my husband, Joe Avarista, and children Meagan Roberts, Archie Roberts, Dorie Roberts, and her husband Luis Reis, form the very foundation of my life.

Finally, I want to thank my patients who are my best teachers, my inspiration, and my exemplars of fortitude, strength, perseverance, and patience.

Introduction

If you are reading this book, chances are excellent that you, or someone you love, is taking a medicine to either prevent or treat heart disease. The word *medicine* is derived from Latin. The Latin word for physician is *medicus* and the word *medicina* means healing. Hopefully, if your doctor prescribes a medicine, she or he is trying to bring about healing. She will have carefully weighed the possible risks versus the possible benefits (what is called the *risk/benefit ratio*) and will have decided that the medicine she has in mind is more likely to help you than harm you. Prescribing medicines is not something that a conscientious physician does lightly. Practicing physicians have all known patients who have had side effects from medications, some of them serious or even fatal. (Though a fatal drug reaction is uncommon, it certainly grabs media attention.)

Ideally your physician will give you specific instructions on how and when to take the medicine and will tell you what the possible side effects are. He also will ask you about any other medicine you might be on to avoid giving you a drug that could interact adversely with one you're already taking. He might tell you about certain foods you need to avoid—or to eat more of—while you are on the medicine. He will give you a chance to ask questions and voice concerns.

Here is a brief word about side effects using headache as an example. There are certainly medicines that can cause a headache, but just because you experience a headache while taking a medicine, it does not necessarily mean that you are having a side effect. The headache may be completely coincidental. Several years ago, a patient whom I had treated for many years, developed a headache. He went to his primary care physician who promptly stopped one of his high blood pressure medicines, which had headache as a possible side effect (despite the fact that the patient had been taking it without a headache for many years). Needless to say his headache did not improve and tests subsequently revealed a brain tumor. Not all examples are this dramatic. However, I've had patients stop taking medicines because they thought they were having side effects when in fact their symptoms were coming from the condition I put them on medicine for in the first place!

Nausea is another symptom that is listed as a possible side effect for just about any medicine you can name. This does not mean, however, that because you experience nausea after taking a medicine it is a side effect. It **may** be, but it could also be the onset of a stomach flu, a gall bladder attack, a heart attack, or any number of other conditions that have nothing to do with your new prescription. It is vital that you discuss any symptom you think may be a side effect with your physician and not simply stop taking the prescribed medicine. Many side effects are mild and resolve on their own, as your body adjusts to the medicine.

In this guide, the most likely side effects and the most potentially dangerous side effects of each medicine will be discussed; however, not every single symptom that has ever been reported by anyone taking the drug is covered. Doing so would make this guide too heavy to carry.

More and more people are becoming computer literate and often, when prescribed a new medicine, will search the Internet for information, especially if they feel their doctor has not fully explained the reasons for taking this new medicine or its possible risks and side effects. Although there are helpful, reputable Web sites with information about prescription and over-the-counter drugs (for example, www.healthfinder.gov and www.fda.gov), there also are others that have information which is biased, misleading, or both. Again, do not stop taking a medicine if you experience what you believe is a side effect (with the exception of the serious allergic reaction mentioned later) without discussing it first with your physician.

Some medicines should not be stopped abruptly. Obviously, if you start a new medicine and you shortly break out in total-body hives, feel weak, or have trouble breathing, these are symptoms of a serious allergic reaction and you need to call 911 and get to the nearest emergency room. For example, abruptly stopping beta-blocker medicines (often prescribed for angina or high blood pressure) may lead to a heart attack or stroke. These and some other medicines need to be tapered slowly to avoid problems.

Here is another word, this one about "natural remedies." I've had patients tell me that they don't want to take drugs, that they want to take natural remedies. They then sometimes show me bottles of nonprescription (but often very expensive) herbs, vitamins, natural hormones, tonics, supplements, gels, and the like. However, because these items (unlike prescription medicines) are not regulated by the Food and Drug Administration (FDA), their manufacturers can make claims about their efficacy without any scientific back up in the way of proof. The remedies may not even contain the ingredients listed on the bottle, and their manufacture is not regulated by the FDA, as is the manufacture of prescription drugs.

I am not implying that Mother Nature does not provide us with substances that can cure disease or alleviate symptoms. After all, digitalis, one of the oldest cardiac medicines is derived from the foxglove (*Digitalis purpura* to give it its botanical name). Aspirin-type medicines were first derived from extracts of white willow bark (*Salix alba vulgaris*; hence the chemical name for aspirin, acetylsalicylic acid), which was used to treat fever for centuries. Quinine, used to treat malaria, is derived from the cinchona tree bark. All drugs, whether "manmade" or "natural," are chemicals, just as all of us are walking, talking chemical soups. Prescription drugs are made up of chemicals just as natural remedies are made up of chemicals. The difference is that with the prescription drug, the active ingredient has undergone testing to prove that it is effective, the label must accurately describe the dose, and the factory where it is manufactured is subject to inspections by the FDA. None of these holds true for natural remedies. I tell my patients who insist on taking them that they are very brave, because they really don't have a clue what they are actually ingesting. Not only that, they are taking a risk that something in the natural remedy will interact with something in their prescription medicines and cause an adverse reaction.

I have tried in this book to provide an accurate, up-to-date guide to the cardiac medicines that are currently prescribed in the United States. I have confined the content to drugs that can be taken by mouth, through the skin, and in one case as a nasal spray. There are other cardiac medicines that can only be given by intravenous or intramuscular injection but they will not be discussed in this guide.

I believe that a well-informed patient is more likely to comply with the doctor's recommendations, and when doctors and patients work together, the results are more satisfactory than when the two are at cross purposes. In achieving health, as in every other endeavor, ignorance is **not** bliss. I hope this book will expand your knowledge and help you maintain your heart health.

CHAPTER 1

Preventing Heart Disease

The most common form of heart disease in the world is caused by atherosclerosis. The term *atherosclerosis* is derived from two Greek words: *athera* which means porridge or gruel and *scleros* which means hard. The term was coined by early pathologists who looked at diseased arteries and thought that what is now referred to as "plaque" looked like hard porridge. The process of forming this atherosclerotic plaque often begins in childhood, especially in countries like the United States where people eat a diet that is high in saturated or animal fat.

Not long after World War II, the U.S. government decided to fund a study to determine what was causing an alarming increase in deaths from heart disease. The study investigators were charged with learning the risk factors for the development of atherosclerosis. A *risk factor* is any substance, characteristic, or action that increases the risk of developing the disease in question. In order to ascertain the risk factors for atherosclerotic cardiovascular disease (ASCVD), two thirds of the adult population of Framingham, Massachusetts, between the ages of 30 and 62 agreed to answer detailed questionnaires, have blood drawn, and come in for follow-up testing every 2 years. Over the ensuing 60-plus years, the Framingham Study contributed immensely to an understanding of the risk factors for ASCVD. It turns out that a staggering 80 to 90 percent of ASCVD is preventable—and of the several risk factors that were discovered, only two cannot be changed. One is your age; the older you get, the more your risk for ASCVD increases. You cannot modify your age. You can lie about it but that doesn't modify it. The other nonmodifiable risk factor is your family history. You might wish that you were born into a different family, or had a different set of genes, but at least today, wishing won't make it happen.

However, all of the other risk factors for ASCVD are either modifiable or completely avoidable. They include high blood pressure, abnormal levels of cholesterol and triglycerides (also called blood lipids), smoking, diabetes, obesity, and sedentary life style. Of these, smoking is completely avoidable, but for those who are addicted to nicotine, there are new medicines that are effective in helping to cure smokers of their craving. Diabetes is another very potent risk factor for ASCVD but it too is largely avoidable by leading a heart healthy lifestyle. To prevent diabetes, there are no medicines that are as effective as regular exercise and maintaining a normal body weight by sensible eating. The rest of this chapter will discuss drugs used to treat high blood pressure, abnormal lipid levels, and nicotine addiction.

MEDICINES TO TREAT HIGH BLOOD PRESSURE

High blood pressure or hypertension is a very common risk factor for developing heart disease. When your blood pressure is measured, there are two numbers that are determined. The higher number or "systolic" pressure is the pressure in the arteries when the heart is contracting. Remember that your heart is a muscular pump and its job is to pump blood around the body. The lower number or "diastolic" pressure is the pressure in the arteries when the heart is relaxed. Both of these numbers are important and if either is elevated, you are at increased risk of developing ASCVD. However, in people who are older than 50 years of age, a high systolic blood pressure is a stronger risk factor than a high diastolic blood pressure. The units used to measure blood pressure are millimeters of mercury (mm Hg), and refer to the height to which a column of mercury can be raised by the pressure in the arteries.

There have been multiple well-designed studies that have proven beyond a shadow of a doubt that lowering high blood pressure lowers the risk of developing heart disease. Luckily, there are also a multitude of medicines that are effective in treating hypertension. The likelihood that you will develop high blood pressure increases with age. In fact, past the age of 60, the majority of people in this country have high blood pressure. High blood pressure is more common is some ethnic groups, such as African Americans, than others. Sometimes high blood pressure is caused by other conditions but most, an estimated 93 to 95 percent, is what doctors call "essential" or "primary," meaning we don't know why it occurs. Five to 7 percent are termed "secondary" because there is another condition that is causing the high blood pressure.

Some conditions that are associated with hypertension include an overactive thyroid, blockage in a kidney artery, chronic kidney disease, certain rare tumors that secrete hormones that raise blood pressure, obesity, sleep apnea, and diets high in sodium (salt). A family history of hypertension also increases your chances of developing the condition as do smoking and excessive alcohol intake. Hypertension can be a side effect of certain medications, such as oral contraceptives, decongestants, or some herbal supplements. If you are diagnosed with high blood pressure, your physician may order tests to determine if you have primary or secondary hypertension.

For adults, optimal blood pressure is defined as being less than 120/80 mm Hg. Normal blood pressure is defined as less than 130/85 mm Hg and high normal blood pressure is defined as 130 to 139/85 to 89 mm Hg. Hypertension is often divided into three stages. Stage 1 refers to blood pressures between 140 to 159/90 to 99 mm Hg. Stage 2 refers to blood pressures between 160 to 179/100 to 109 mm Hg. Stage 3 refers to blood pressures of 180/110 mm Hg or higher. The risk of developing cardiovascular disease (CVD) begins to increase at a blood pressure above 115/75 and risk doubles with every additional 20/10 mm Hg increase in blood pressure.

Except in cases of severe high blood pressure, the first step in treating mild degrees of hypertension is lifestyle modification. Smoking cessation is imperative. A diet high in fruits and vegetables and low in salt will often bring a slightly elevated blood pressure back into the normal range. Weight loss for those who are overweight and regular aerobic exercise (at least 30 minutes most days of the week) also are beneficial. If you drink more than two 8-ounce glasses of wine, 2 ounces of liquor, or 24 ounces of beer daily, you will be asked to lower these amounts or stop alcohol completely if your blood pressure is still out of control.

When lifestyle changes are not enough to achieve normal levels after 3 to 6 months, your doctor will prescribe medicines to treat your high blood pressure. The tables of medications that follow the descriptions of each drug give the range of daily doses. Some of these medicines can be taken once a day; others need to be taken more than once a day. Always be sure that you understand how your physician or nurse practitioner wants you to take your medicine. Your pharmacist also will provide you with information about dosage schedules and whether you should take your pills on an empty stomach or with meals.

Diuretics

The panel of experts called the Joint National Committee (JNC) on Prevention, Detection, Evaluation, and Treatment of High Blood Pressure came out with revised recommendations about hypertension treatment in 2003. This report, called the JNC 7 recommended that *thiazide diuretics* be used either alone or in combination with other drugs in the treatment of most patients with uncomplicated hypertension. Thiazide diuretics work by increasing the excretion of sodium by the kidneys. They also may cause loss of potassium, which can be a serious side effect, potentially causing abnormal heart rhythms and muscle damage. Potassium is a chemical found in the blood that is important for maintaining muscle strength and for stabilizing the heart rhythm. The kidneys tightly regulate levels of potassium because having too high a level or too low a level of potassium both are very dangerous.

Your potassium level should be checked periodically while you are taking a thiazide diuretic, particularly when you first start the medicine, or if you have any illness likely to lower your potassium, such as significant vomiting or diarrhea. Symptoms of low blood potassium include muscle weakness or cramps, dizziness, nausea, and palpitations.

Another potential side effect of thiazide diuretics that is not related to potassium level is erectile dysfunction. Thiazide diuretics also may increase the level of blood sugar, cholesterol, triglycerides, and uric acid, the last of which can lead to attacks of gout. In people who are also taking digitalis, loss of potassium may be particularly dangerous so people on both a thiazide diuretic and digitalis may need to take potassium supplements. Sometimes thiazide diuretics can bring on an attack of pancreatitis (inflamed pancreas) in people who have a history of that dis-

Table 1–1 Thiazide and Thiazide-like Diuretics

Drug (Trade Name)	Dosage Range (mg/d)
Chlorothiazide (Diuril®)	500–2,000
Hydrochlorothiazide (Hydrodiuril®)	12.5–50
Chlorthalidone (Hygroton®)	12.5–50
Indapamide (Lozol®)	1.25–5.0
Metolazone (Zaroxolyn®)	2.5–5.0
Polythiazide (Renese®)	1.0–4.0
Bendroflumethazide (Naturetin®)	2.5–10

order. More rarely a drop in white and red blood cell counts occurs in people taking these medications. As with any medicine, allergic reactions can occur, most often in the form of a rash.

When the results of several large studies of the use of thiazides to treat hypertension were pooled and analyzed, patients treated with these medicines had a higher likelihood of developing diabetes than patients taking other classes of medicines called angiotensin-converting enzyme inhibitors or angiotensin receptor blockers.

Thiazide diuretics usually are taken once a day. Table 1–1 lists the most commonly prescribed thiazide diuretics with their generic and trade names and usual dosage range.

Because of their propensity to cause loss of potassium, thiazide diuretics often are combined with a class of medicines called *potassium-sparing diuretics*. Table 1–2 lists the most common potassium-sparing diuretics, followed by some of the available combinations of potassium-sparing diuretics with other diuretics.

Spironolactone and eplerenone are more effective in lowering blood pressure than triamterene or amiloride, neither of which has any significant effect on blood

Table 1–2 Potassium-sparing Diuretics and Combination Diuretics

Drug (Trade Name)	Dosage Range (mg/d)
Spironolactone (Aldactone®)	12.5–50
Triamterene (Dyrenium®)	25–50
Amiloride (Midamor®)	5–10
Eplerenone (Inspra®)	50–100
Spironolactone/Hydrochlorothiazide (Aldactazide®)	25/25
Triamterene/Hydrochlorothiazide (Dyazide, Maxide®)	37.5–75/25
Amiloride/Hydrochlorothiazide (Moduretic®)	5/50

pressure when taken alone. Potassium-sparing diuretics may cause dangerous elevations in blood potassium levels, particularly in people with kidney disease or people who are taking certain other classes of blood pressure medications, ACE (angiotensin-converting enzyme) inhibitors, and angiotensin receptor blockers. Your physician should monitor your potassium level when you are taking these diuretics.

Spironolactone sometimes causes another side effect that is particularly bothersome in men: breast enlargement, what doctors refer to as *gynecomastia*. It also can raise levels of digoxin, a form of digitalis, in people taking both medicines.

Finally, there are diuretics that are called *loop diuretics* because they act on a portion of the kidney called the Loop of Henle. These medicines are more potent than the diuretics just listed and usually cause the excretion of more urine. They therefore are more apt to lead to dehydration and low potassium levels. When used in high doses, loop diuretics sometimes can lead to ringing in the ears, vertigo, and hearing loss.

Table 1–3 lists the loop diuretics with their usual dosage ranges.

ACE Inhibitors

The abbreviation ACE stands for angiotensin-converting enzyme. Medicines that inhibit the action of this enzyme dilate blood vessels and lower blood pressure. The way they work is somewhat complicated but what follows is a brief, simplified explanation.

Our bodies have evolved something called the renin-angiotensin-aldosterone system (RAAS) that is called into play when our blood pressure drops; for example, if we become dehydrated or lose a significant amount of blood. In such situations, the kidney releases a substance called *renin*, which then cleaves a protein manufactured by the liver called *angiotensinogen*, turning it into a substance called *angiotensin I*. Another enzyme, *angiotensin-converting enzyme*, then cleaves angiotensin I, forming angiotensin II which has a powerful effect on arteries, causing them to constrict. Angiotensin II also has other effects. It stimulates overgrowth of muscle fibers in the heart (what doctors call *left ventricular hypertrophy* or LVH) and it stimulates the release of two hormones, one from the adrenal gland and one from the pituitary gland. The hormone from the adrenal gland is called

Table 1–3 Loop Diuretics

Drug (Trade) Name	Dosage Range (mg/d)
Furosemide (Lasix®)	20–80
Bumetanide (Bumex®)	0.5–2
Torsemide (Demadex®)	5–10

aldosterone. Aldosterone causes the kidney to retain salt (sodium chloride) and water and to excrete potassium. The other hormone, which is released by the pituitary gland, is called *vasopressin*. Vasopressin also is called *anti-diuretic hormone* or ADH, and it causes the kidney to retain water. The net result of all of this is to increase the blood volume and to increase blood pressure.

ACE inhibitors work by interfering with the formation of angiotensin II from angiotensin I. Becuase they also interfere with the release of aldosterone, they can cause increases in blood potassium, particularly in people who have diseased kidneys. In people with chronic kidney disease, ACE inhibitors can cause worsening of kidney function. However, this class of medicines has been shown to protect the kidneys from the ravages of diabetes and are widely prescribed for this purpose.

ACE inhibitors can harm and even kill a fetus, so they should not be prescribed to pregnant women. Sometimes people develop a dry cough when they take ACE inhibitors. Although this is bothersome, it is not dangerous. A more serious side effect is the development of an allergic reaction called *angioedema*. This involves swelling and itching around the mouth and throat and can seriously interfere with breathing. If these symptoms occur, prompt treatment in an emergency room is necessary.

Particularly when taken with diuretics or in people who are dehydrated for whatever reason, ACE inhibitors can cause a marked drop in blood pressure, leading to dizziness or even fainting. ACE inhibitors seem to be less effective in lowering blood pressures in blacks than whites and are more apt to cause angioedema in blacks.

Table 1–4 lists the commonly prescribe ACE inhibitors and their usual doses. Captopril and moexipril should be taken an hour before meals. The other ACE inhibitors can be taken without regard to meals.

ACE inhibitors often are combined with diuretics. Table 1–5 lists some of the commonly prescribed medicines that contain both an ACE inhibitor and a di-

Table 1–4 ACE Inhibitors

Drug (Trade Name)	Dosage Range (mg/d)
Benazepril (Lotensin®)	5–40
Captopril (Capoten®)	50–300
Enalapril (Vasotec®)	5–40
Fosinopril (Monopril®)	10–80
Lisinopril (Zestril, Prinivil®)	5–40
Moexipril (Univasc®)	7.5–30
Perindopril (Aceon®)	4–16
Quinapril (Accupril®)	10–80
Ramipril (Altace®)	2.5–20
Trandolapril (Mavik®)	1–4

Table 1–5 ACE Inhibitor/Diuretic Combinations

Drug (Trade Name)	Dosage Range (mg/d)
Benazepril/HCTZ (Lotensin HCT®)	5/6.25–20/25
Captopril/HCTZ (Capozide®)	25/15–50/25
Lisinopril/HCTZ (Zestoretic, Prinizide®)	10/12.5–20/25
Moexipril/HCTZ (Uniretic®)	7.5/12.5–15/25
Quinapril/HCTZ (Accuretic®)	10/12.5–20/25
Enalapril/HCTZ (Vaseretic®)	5/12.5–10/25

uretic. The most commonly used diuretic in these combinations is hydrochlorothiazide, which will be abbreviated as HCTZ.

Angiotensin Receptor Blockers

Angiotensin receptor blockers (ARBs) also interfere with the RAAS but they do so at a different point than do ACE inhibitors; they block the uptake of angiotensin II onto receptors in the smooth muscle in the walls of blood vessels. Because angiotensin II causes arteries to constrict, blocking this action causes arteries to dilate, lowering blood pressure. Like ACE inhibitors, ARBs can cause high blood levels of potassium, especially in people with kidney disease, but they are much less likely to have cough as a side effect—and like ACE inhibitors, ARBs can cause worsening kidney failure in people with diseased kidneys, but protect diabetics from developing kidney failure. ARBs can also cause harm to a fetus so they should not be used by pregnant women. Table 1–6 lists the commonly prescribed ARBs. ARBs can be combined with diuretics, and Table 1–7 lists the commonly prescribed ARB/diuretic combinations.

Table 1–6 Angiotensin Receptor Blockers (ARB's)

Drug (Trade Name)	Dosage Range (mg/d)
Candesartan (Atacand®)	8–32
Eprosartan (Teveten®)	400–800
Irbesartan (Avapro®)	150–300
Losartan (Cozaar®)	25–100
Olmesartan (Benicar®)	20–40
Telmisartan (Micardis®)	20–80
Valsartan (Diovan®)	80–320

Table 1–7 ARB/diuretic combinations

Drug (Trade Name)	Dosage Range (mg/d)
Candesartan/HCTZ (Atacand HCT®)	16/12.5–32/12.5
Eprosartan/HCTZ (Teveten HCT®)	600/12.5–600/25
Irbesartan/HCTZ (Avalide®)	150/12.5–300/25
Losartan/HCTZ (Hyzaar®)	50/12.5–100/25
Olmesartan/HCTZ (Benicar HCT®)	20/12.5–40/25
Telmisartan/HCTZ (Micardis HCT®)	40/12.5–80/25
Valsartan/HCTZ (Diovan HCT®)	80/12.5–320/25

Beta-Blockers

Beta-blockers have been in widespread use to treat high blood pressure for several decades. To understand how they work, you need to know a bit about the body's nervous system. The nervous system can be classified in two ways: one based on anatomy, the other based on function. Anatomically, the nervous system consists of the brain and spinal cord (the *central nervous system* or CNS) and the *peripheral nervous system*, consisting of the nerves (also called neurons) that travel to and from the central nervous system to every organ in the body. The nervous system also can be divided functionally into two parts called the *somatic* and the *autonomic*.

The somatic nervous system is under our conscious control. It consists of sensory nerves that receive information from the world around us and motor neurons that control movement. An example of the somatic nervous system in operation is the common experience of getting a paper cut on a finger. Sensory nerves in the skin are stimulated by the injury and the resulting impulse reaches the brain, which sends out impulses to neurons that control the muscles of the arm, prompting us to snatch our hand out of harm's way. In summary, the somatic nervous system receives sensory information from the outside world, brings it to the CNS and controls the skeletal muscles of the body.

For the most part, the autonomic nervous system is not under our conscious control. It consists of neurons that transmit impulses from the CNS to the various organs of the body, such as the heart, liver, skin, and the like, and other neurons that transmit impulses from the peripheral organs to the CNS. The autonomic nervous system affects things like heart rate, perspiration, pupil size, contraction and relaxation of smooth muscles in the bowel, airways and blood vessels, and the release of certain hormones. The autonomic neurons that travel to the CNS can carry pain sensations from the abdominal organs and are important in helping to regulate respiration, pulse rate, and blood pressure.

The autonomic nervous system is subdivided into the *parasympathetic* and the *sympathetic* nervous systems. Most organs have nerve fibers from both of these divisions, and they generally have opposing actions. For example, the parasympathetic nerve fibers going to the heart slow it down, while the sympathetic fibers speed it up. The classic description of the sympathetic nervous system is that it prepares us for "fight or flight" while the parasympathetic nervous system kicks in when it's time to "rest and digest."

When the sympathetic nervous system is activated, chemicals called *catecholamines* are released from nerve endings and are taken up by receptors in, for example, arterial smooth muscle or the muscle fibers in the heart. The two most common catecholamines are *epinephrine* and *norepinephrine* (also called *adrenalin* and *noradrenalin*). Catecholamines are neurotransmitters, which are substances that travel across a gap between neurons (that gap is called a *synapse*) and carry information. In order for that information to be received, the neurotransmitter must be taken up by a receptor on the cell surface.

There are two main types of receptors in the sympathetic nervous system called α (alpha) and β (beta) receptors. Any substance that prevents a chemical from binding to a receptor is called a *blocker* or *antagonist* and any substance that enhances binding to a receptor is called an *agonist*. Therefore, a beta-blocker is a substance that prevents binding to a beta-receptor.

There are different kinds of beta-receptors, one found mainly in the heart, and another found in the smooth muscles of arteries, bronchi (air tubes in the lungs), and the gastrointestinal tract. A medicine that blocks the first type of beta-receptor is called *cardioselective* and the latter is called a *nonselective* beta-blocker. Some beta-blockers also have alpha-blocking activity and some have what is called *intrinsic sympathomimetic activity*; in other words, they both block and stimulate sympathetic activity at the same time.

The beta-blockers, particularly the nonselective ones, can cause wheezing and exacerbate asthma in people with that condition. Beta-blockers also can mask the symptoms of low blood sugar and so diabetics, particularly those on insulin, must be made aware of this. In people with certain types of blockage in the electrical conducting system of the heart, beta-blockers can lead to marked slowing of the heart rate, so they should be avoided in that situation. Occasionally beta-blockers are associated with fatigue, nightmares, and depression but in many studies, these complaints were no more frequent in people taking beta-blockers than in those taking placebo or "dummy" pills. Rarely, beta-blockers can lead to hair loss, erectile dysfunction, and increases in triglycerides, but in general, they are very safe medications.

When the results of several large studies of the use of beta-blockers to treat hypertension were pooled and analyzed, patients treated with these medicines had a higher likelihood of developing diabetes than patients taking ACE inhibitors or ARBs and their use as first-line drugs to treat high blood pressure has fallen out of favor.

Table 1–8 lists some of the commonly prescribed beta-blockers, both cardioselective and nonselective, Table 1–9 lists the beta-blockers with alpha-blocking

Table 1–8 Cardioselective Beta-Blockers

Drug (Trade Name)	Dosage Range (mg/d)
Metoprolol (Lopressor®, Toprol®, Toprol XL®)	25–200
Atenolol (Tenormin®)	25–100
Bisoprolol (Zebeta®)	2.5–20
Betaxolol (Kerlone®)	5–20
Nebivolol (Bystolic®)	5–40
Non-selective beta-blockers	
Propranolol (Inderal®, Inderal LA®)	40–240
Nadolol (Corgard®)	40–320
Timolol (Blocadren®)	20–60

activity and those that have intrinsic sympathomimetic activity, and Table 1–10 lists some of the beta-blocker/diuretic combinations available in the United States.

Calcium Channel Blockers

Calcium channel blockers (CCBs) work by affecting the flow of calcium through microscopic pores in cells, including muscle cells in the heart and blood vessels, causing these muscles to contract less strongly or relax. When the muscle cells in the walls of arteries relax, this leads to a drop in blood pressure.

CCBs are divided into two classes: *non-dihydropyridines* and *dihydropyridines.* The former class exerts effects on the strength of contraction of cardiac muscle and the propagation of the electrical impulses that control the heart rate. For this reason, CCBs of this type can cause slowing of the heart rate, and a decrease in the strength of heart muscle contraction. The former effect may be beneficial, for ex-

Table 1–9 Beta-Blockers with Alpha-Blocking Activity

Drug (Trade Name)	Dosage Range (mg/d)
Carvedilol (Coreg®, Coreg CR®)	12.5–50, 20–80
Labetalol (Normodyne®, Trandate®)	200–2400
Beta-Blockers with Intrinsic Sympathomimetic Activity	
Pindolol (Visken®)	10–60
Acebutolol (Sectral®)	200–1200
Penbutolol (Levatol®)	20–40

Table 1–10 Beta blocker/diuretic combinations

Drug (Trade Name)	Dosage Range (mg/d)
Atenolol/chlorthalidone (Tenoretic®)	50/25–100/25
Timolol/HCTZ (Timolide®)	10/25–20/50
Bisoprolol/HCTZ (Ziac®)	2.5/6.25–20/12.5
Propranolol LA/HCTZ (Inderide LA®)	40/25–160/50
Metoprolol/HCTZ (Lopressor HCT®)	50/25–100/50
Nadolol/bendroflumethiazide (Corzide®)	40/5–80/5

ample, when these drugs are used to treat fast heart rhythms (called *tachycardias* or *tachyarrhythmias*), but at times, the heart rate can drop too much and cause symptoms such as dizziness or even fainting. This type of CCB also can cause increased shortness of breath in people who have congestive heart failure due to weakened heart muscle, so, in general, they should not be used in that condition.

The dihydropyridine CCBs affect predominantly the smooth muscle in the arterial wall and do not affect the pulse rate or strength of heart muscle contraction directly. The most common side effects of the dihydropyridine CCBs are headache and swelling (edema) of the ankles. Women tend to experience edema more often than men do. Edema is less likely to occur in people taking this type of CCB if they also are taking an ACE inhibitor or an ARB. Much less commonly, patients report sexual dysfunction while taking CCBs. The CCBs, especially when combined with a diuretic, are particularly effective in the treatment of hypertension in African Americans.

Table 1–11 lists the dihydropyridine and nondihydropyridine calcium channel blockers available in the United States. Only the long-acting forms of the CCBs are listed because short-acting preparations are not generally used to treat high blood pressure.

Combinations of CCBs and ACE inhibitors also are available to treat high blood pressure. Many people will require more than one type of antihypertensive to achieve a normal blood pressure. Combining two medicines in one pill often lowers the cost and avoids the increased likelihood of side effects that occurs when medicines are pushed to their highest dose. In 2007 the FDA approved a combination pill incorporating a CCB and an ARB.

Table 1–12 lists the combinations of a CCB and an ACE inhibitor or ARB available in this country.

Alpha-Blockers

Earlier it was mentioned that the sympathetic nervous system has two main types of receptors called alpha and beta receptors. Alpha receptors occur in the smooth muscle found in the walls of arteries, and when they are activated, the arteries constrict, raising blood pressure. Medicines that block the alpha receptors lower blood

Table 1–11 Dihydropyridine CCB's

Drug (Trade Name)	Dosage Range (mg/d)
Amlodipine (Norvasc®)	2.5–10
Felodipine (Plendil®)	2.5–10
Isradipine (DynaCirc CR®)	5.0–20
Nicardipine (Cardene SR®)	60–120
Nifedipine (Adalat CC, Procardia XL®)	30–90
Nisoldipine (Sular®)	10–40

Non-dihydropyridine CCB's

Drug (Trade) Name	Dosage Range mg/d
Diltiazem (Cardizem CD®, Dilacor XR®, Tiazac®)	120–480
Verapamil (Calan SR®, Isoptin SR®, Covera HS®)	120–480

pressure. Because they relax smooth muscle throughout the body, they also are used to treat other conditions, such as an enlarged prostate and Raynaud's disease, a condition in which small arteries in the fingers constrict on exposure to cold temperatures, sometimes severely enough to cause gangrene.

The most common side effect of alpha-blockers is dizziness. Especially when this type of medicine is taken for the first time, there may be a pronounced drop in blood pressure leading to dizziness and in some cases, even fainting. This is most often apt to occur when going from a horizontal or sitting position to a vertical position. Other common side effects are headache and awareness of heart pounding. Alpha-blockers are rarely used as first-line therapy for high blood pressure; in fact, one study of a large group of people with hypertension found that those treated with alpha-blockers over a long term had a higher chance of developing heart failure than those treated with other agents.

Table 1–13 lists the alpha-blockers and a combination alpha-blocker/diuretic used to treat hypertension in the United States.

Table 1–12 CCB/ACE Inhibitor or ARB Combinations

Drug (Trade Name)	Dosage Range (mg/d)
Amlodipine/benazepril (Lotrel®)	2.5/10–10/40
Verapamil/trandolapril (Tarka®)	2/180–4/240
Felodipine/enalapril (Lexxel®)	5/5–10/10
Amlodipine/valsartan (Exforge®)	5/160–10/320

Table 1–13 Alpha-Blockers

Drug (Trade Name)	Dosage Range (mg/d)
Doxazosin (Cardura®)	1–16
Prazosin (Minipress®)	2–20
Terazosin (Hytrin®)	1–20

Alpha-Blocker/Diuretic Combination	
Prazosin/polythiazide (Minizide®)	1/0.5–5/0.5

There are two other classes of medicines that are used to treat hypertension. They are not used as first-line drugs but are added to other medicines to achieve blood pressure goals. The first are called *direct vasodilators* and the second are called *centrally acting drugs* (because they are considered to act on the central nervous system).

The direct vasodilators can cause flushing, rapid heart rate, headache, fluid retention, and in the case of minoxidil, increased hair growth (so it's sometimes prescribed to treat hair loss). In the case of hydralazine, a rare but potentially serious side effect is the development of the disease called *lupus erythematosis*. Table 1–14 lists the direct vasodilators and their usual daily dosage range along with a combination pill of this class.

The centrally acting blood pressure medicines, with the exception of clonidine, are rarely used today. They were among the first agents used clinically to treat hypertension, but because of limited efficacy and side effects and the discovery of more effective drugs, they have fallen out of favor. These medicines must be taken for a few weeks before the effect on blood pressure is optimized. Drowsiness is the most common side effect, especially in the first few weeks of use. Dry mouth, erectile dysfunction, fluid retention, and constipation also can occur with centrally acting blood pressure medicines.

Clonidine should not be stopped abruptly because a rebound marked elevation in blood pressure may occur. Except in the case of a serious allergic reaction, clonidine should be tapered over several days if it needs to be discontinued and your

Table 1–14 Direct Vasodilators/Vasodilator/diuretic combination

Drug (Trade Name)	Dosage Range (mg/d)
Hydralazine (Apresoline®)	40–200
Minoxidil (Loniten®)	2.5–80
Hydralazine/HCTZ (Apresazide®)	25/25–100/50

Table 1–15 Centrally Acting Blood Pressure Medicines

Drug (Trade Name)	Dosage Range (mg/d)
Clonidine (Catapres®)	0.1–0.8
Clonidine Patch (CatapresTTS®, applied weekly)	0.1–0.6
Methyldopa (Aldomet®)	250–2000
Reserpine (Serpalan®)	0.05–0.25
Guanfacine (Tenex®)	0.5–2

Centrally Acting Blood Pressure Medicine Combinations

Drug (Trade Name)	Dosage Range (mg/d)
Clonidine/chlorthalidone (Combipres®)	0.1/15–0.3/15
Methyldopa/HCTZ (Aldoril®)	250/15–500/50
Reserpine/chlorothiazide (Diupres®)	0.125/250–0.25/500
Reserpine/HCTZ (Hydropres®)	0.125/25–0.125/50

doctor should monitor you carefully. Clonidine comes in both pill and patch form (the latter is applied once a week to the skin). Stomach ulcers are a possible side effect of reserpine. Abnormalities of liver blood tests and rarely, anemia can occur with methyldopa. Table 1–15 lists the centrally acting blood pressure medicines and some combinations with thiazide diuretics.

Finally, in 2007 the FDA approved the first new antihypertension medicine in more than 10 years. It acts by directly inhibiting renin, the enzyme released by the kidney that cleaves angiotensinogen, forming angiotensin I (see earlier in this chapter). Called aliskiren (trade name Tekturna®), in clinical trials, it was effective in lowering blood pressure in people with mild to moderate hypertension, although it was slightly less effective in blacks than in whites or Asians. Side effects generally were mild; the most common being diarrhea. Cough and rash were less common, and angioedema was rarer still. Like other medicines that affect the RAAS, aliskiren should not be taken by pregnant women because of the potential for harm or even death of the fetus. The full effect of aliskiren on blood pressure may take up to two weeks to achieve. Table 1–16 lists this new high blood pressure medicine and its usual daily dose.

As you can see, today's doctor has a large number of medicines at his or her disposal to lower blood pressure and prevent the ravages that hypertension causes when it is left untreated. Preventing strokes, heart attacks, heart failure, and kidney failure are all proven benefits of treating hypertension. If you are intolerant of one class of medicine, your physician has a number of other choices to help you achieve your blood pressure goal. It is up to you, however, to limit your alcohol and salt intake, avoid smoking and second-hand smoke, eat lots of fruits and vegetables (five-to-seven servings a day), exercise regularly, and avoid packing on the pounds.

MEDICINES TO TREAT ABNORMAL BLOOD LIPIDS

Sometimes when I ask a new patient why he or she was referred to me, I get the response: "I have cholesterol." Well, we all have cholesterol; in fact, we couldn't live without it. *Cholesterol* is a waxy substance that cannot dissolve in water (and our blood is mostly water). It is an important component of cell walls, is required for the synthesis of bile acids (necessary in digestion of food), and is a building block for several hormones, including the reproductive hormones. The cholesterol in the blood comes from two sources: the liver makes it and we absorb it from food.

Because cholesterol is insoluble in water, it circulates in the blood, bound to special proteins called *lipoproteins* (*lipos* means fat in Greek), which make the cholesterol soluble. The lipoproteins are classified according to their density, or weight per unit volume. Going from lowest to highest density, the lipoproteins are:

- Chylomicrons
- Very low density lipoprotein (VLDL)
- Low density lipoprotein (LDL)
- Intermediate density lipoprotein (IDL)
- High density lipoprotein (HDL)
- Lp(a) (usually referred to as "Lp little a")

You are probably aware of the terms "*good*" cholesterol and "*bad*" cholesterol. These refer to HDL cholesterol (HDL-C) and LDL cholesterol (LDL-C). If you have trouble remembering which is which, remember H stands for healthy and L stands for lousy.

HDL-C acts as a scavenger and can actually remove cholesterol from the walls of arteries, bringing it back to the liver where it can be metabolized and excreted. HDL-C also has antioxidant and anti-inflammatory properties, both of which are considered to protect against the development of atherosclerosis.

The *plaque* that builds up in diseased arteries is a complex substance. Plaque contains not only cholesterol but also specialized white blood cells called *macrophages*, smooth muscle cells, various proteins, and sometimes calcium. When an artery is damaged (for example, by any of the poisons in cigarette smoke), LDL-C which has been oxidized (oxidation is the process of combining with oxygen; probably the most common example is the rusting of iron) gets into the arterial wall. White blood cells called *macrophages* "swallow" the LDL-C becoming swollen in the process. They then are called *foam cells*. As plaques grow, they begin to impinge on the opening or lumen of the artery. If plaques become inflamed, they can rupture, releasing clot-promoting material into the bloodstream. When plaques rupture and clots form blocking a heart artery, the result is a heart attack, or death of heart muscle due to interruption of its blood supply. When this happens in the brain, the result is a stroke. Therefore, a key to preventing a buildup of plaque in an artery is maintaining low levels of LDL-C and high levels of HDL-C.

VLDL contains most of the other important blood lipid, called *triglycerides*. Triglycerides are found in dietary fat and they also are produced by the body in response to diets high in carbohydrates. When fats are digested, they are repackaged in the intestines into the lightest lipoproteins, the chylomicrons. In the capillaries of muscle and fatty tissue, chylomicrons are broken down into molecules called *free fatty acids*. These either can be used by muscle cells for energy or stored in the body in fat (adipose) tissue. Fatty acids also are taken up by the liver where they are repackaged as VLDL.

Lp(a) is a modified form of LDL-C that is made in the liver. When it is elevated, it appears to be a risk factor for the development of atherosclerosis.

Abnormal levels of cholesterol and triglycerides may be due to an inherited disorder, or can be due to our diets, various diseases, and certain medications. The diseases that may be associated with abnormal blood lipids include cirrhosis, obstructive liver disease, kidney disease, diabetes, and hypothyroidism (underactive thyroid). Diets high in saturated and trans fats (partially hydrogenated vegetables oils; found in many processed and fast foods) raise levels of LDL-C. Diets high in carbohydrates or consumption of alcohol increase triglyceride levels. Some of the drugs that can cause abnormal blood lipids include retroviral drugs used to treat AIDS, beta blockers, thiazide diuretics, estrogen, and steroids. Before treating you with medicine, your doctor will want to be sure that none of these factors are contributing to your abnormal lipid values.

In the early 1970s when I was a young researcher at the National Heart Lung and Blood Institute (NHLBI), I worked at the lipid metabolism branch under Dr. Robert Levy who, along with Dr. Donald Fredrickson, published an article in 1967 in the *New England Journal of Medicine*, describing and classifying disorders of blood fats. Our group at the NHLBI was charged with designing and implementing studies to determine the prevalence of lipid disorders in the United States and to prove whether lowering high cholesterol would lower the risk of developing signs and symptoms of coronary artery disease (CAD).

At that time, there were only a few medicines available to treat lipid disorders. One, called clofibrate (Atromid®), worked mainly to lower triglyerides and had no significant effect on levels of LDL-C, although in some patients, LDL-C actually increased. Another was the female hormone, estrogen. Estrogen taken by mouth increases levels of HDL-C and lowers levels of LDL-C. Also available in the 1970s was niacin, a B vitamin, which, in large doses, lowers triglycerides and raises HDL-C but does not have a very large effect on LDL-C levels. Finally, the only medicine back in the 1970s that actually lowered LDL-C levels by a significant amount was a medicine called cholestyramine.

Bile Acid Sequestrants

Cholestyramine belongs to a class of medicines called *bile acid sequestrants.* Bile acids form in the intestine from cholesterol and they are important in the digestion and absorption of fats. Bile acid sequestrants bind to bile acids, thereby increasing their excretion, which leads to a lowering of cholesterol and LDL-C levels in the blood.

The problem with cholestyramine in its early days was that it came as a gritty powder that had to be mixed with something like orange juice to disguise the taste, and taken three or four times a day. To make matters worse, it frequently caused constipation and flatulence (the medical term for the common fart). Despite this, cholestyramine was used in the very first study that showed a benefit of lowering high levels of LDL-C. Called the Lipid Research Clinics Intervention Trial, the investigators found a 19 percent reduction in the relative risk of heart attack and cardiac death over seven years in a group of healthy middle-aged men with high LDL-Cs, half of whom got cholestyramine and half of whom got a placebo. Unfortunately, because there were no women in the study, it is unclear if the benefit of this therapy applies to women as well as men, and to this date, researchers have no clinical trial proof that treatment with bile acid sequestrants will lower the risk of cardiac events in women. What *can* be said is that they are effective in lowering LDL-C in women, and because they are not absorbed into the body, they can be taken by women who are pregnant or may become pregnant.

Other possible side effects of bile acid sequestrants include abdominal discomfort, nausea, loss of appetite, intestinal obstruction (in children), and interference with the absorption of other medicines or vitamins. Bleeding due to interference with the absorption of vitamin K and rarely night blindness due to interference with the absorption of vitamin A have been reported in people on bile acid sequestrants. It is important to take other medicines at least 1 hour before or four to six hours after bile acid sequestrants to avoid interfering with their absorption. This class of medicine should not be prescribed to people who have high triglyceride levels because an increase in triglycerides in people taking these medicines is quite common.

Bile acids sequestrants are used in a type of cirrhosis called *primary biliary cirrhosis,* because they decrease the itching that occurs in that condition. Table 1–16 lists the bile acid sequestrants available in the United States today.

Table 1–16 Direct Renin Inhibitor

Drug (Trade Name)	Dosage Range (mg/d)
Aliskiren (Tekturna®)	150–300

Table 1–17 Bile Acid Sequestrants

Drug (Trade) Name	Dosage Range (g/d)
Cholestyramine (Questran®, Questran Lite®)	8–16
Colestipol (Colestid®)	2–16
Colesevelam (WelChol®)	2.50–3.75

Cholestyramine powder has been reformulated so that it is more palatable, but it still must be mixed with six ounces of liquid and taken two to four times a day. Taking it dry can cause choking and should not be attempted. The other two bile acid sequestrants, colestipol and colesevelam, are available in pill form. In general, these medicines are taken twice a day with meals although colestipol and colesevelam may be taken once daily. Bile acid sequestrants sometimes are taken in conjunction with other lipid-lowering drugs, for example, statins and niacin. This allows your physician to achieve your lipid goal without increasing the dose of statin or niacin, and thereby increasing the risk of side effects. Table 1–17 lists the bile acid sequestrants available in the United States.

Niacin

Niacin also is called nicotinic acid or vitamin B3. *Vitamins* are molecules that are essential for life but are not manufactured by our bodies. They act to facilitate chemical reactions in the body. For example, all of the B vitamins help to metabolize carbohydrates, converting them into glucose, which is a primary source of energy for the body.

Lack of vitamins in the diet can lead to several diseases. For example, scurvy, a disease in which vitamin C is lacking, causes impaired wound healing, bleeding from the gums and bowel, and, if not treated, death. Rickets is a disease caused by lack of vitamin D and it can cause weak bones, bowed legs, and shortened stature.

Lack of niacin causes pellagra. People with this disease have a scaly skin rash (the term *pellagra* is from two Italian words: *pelle*, skin, and *agra*, bitter), mental confusion, diarrhea, inflamed mucous membranes, dementia, and death. Nowadays, it is seen most frequently in alcoholics or others who eat a very restricted diet.

Niacin interferes with the liver's ability to make triglycerides and reduces the clearance of HDL-C from the blood. These two actions lead to lower triglyceride and higher HDL-C levels, beneficial results which are particularly important in women. Niacin also has a modest LDL-C lowering effect and is one of the few drugs that also decreases Lp(a). Niacin usually is prescribed with another lipid-lowering medication, most commonly a statin, but sometimes a fibrate or bile acid sequestrant.

While the recommended daily allowance of niacin is about 14 to 18 mg, the dose of niacin necessary to improve blood lipids is much higher in the range of 1,500 to 3,000 mg/day. At these doses, niacin often causes flushing, a bothersome but not

Table 1–18 Prescription Sustained Release Niacin and Niacin-Combination Drugs

Drug (Trade) Name	Dosage Range (mg/d)
Niacin (Niaspan®)	1,000–2,000
Niacin/Lovastatin (Advicor®)	500/20–2,000/40

dangerous side effect that tends to diminish over time. Sustained-release forms of niacin are less likely to cause flushing and their use has supplanted that of immediate-release niacin. To further lessen the chance of flushing, your physician will usually instruct you to take a full dose (325 mg) aspirin (or a nonsteroidal anti-inflammatory medicine like ibuprofen) about 30 minutes before taking niacin, and to eat a low-fat snack that includes apples or applesauce with the dose of niacin. (The pectin in apples helps prevent flushing). It is usual to start out with a lower dose, usually 500 mg/d and increase by 500 mg/d each week until the desired dose is achieved.

Other potential side effects of niacin include increases in blood sugar, particularly in people who are diabetic, or prediabetic, increases in uric acid that can lead to gout, acid reflux, stomach ulcers, and increases in liver enzymes. Your doctor will monitor your liver blood tests while you are taking niacin.

Some over-the-counter sustained-release forms of niacin were associated with severe liver damage but prescription sustained-release niacin is safer because its manufacture is subject to better quality control. The FDA regulates prescription drug quality, but not that of dietary supplements or over-the-counter medicines. Table 1–18 lists the prescription sustained-release niacin and niacin-combination drugs available in the United States.

Statins

Statins are the most effective drugs currently available for lowering LDL-C and are the medicines for which researchers have the best evidence of benefit in preventing cardiac events. A short digression here will illustrate what is meant by this.

When physicians and scientists want to determine if a drug is effective, they undertake what is called a *randomized, double-blind, placebo-controlled study*, also known as a *randomized controlled trial* (*RCT*). When they want to determine if a drug prevents a disease or its manifestations, they call that a *prevention trial*. There are two main types of prevention: primary and secondary. A primary prevention trial is performed with people who as best can be determined do not have the disease being studied. A secondary prevention trial is performed with people who already have the disease. They have had an "event" (for example, a heart attack). In that kind of trial, the investigators are trying to determine if the drug being studied lowers the risk of having additional events.

In both primary and secondary prevention trials, the people who agree to participate are randomly assigned to receive either the active drug or a dummy pill called a *placebo*. Every effort is made to ensure that the two groups have a similar level of risk. Their average age will be the same and they will have similar levels of blood lipids, blood pressure, smoking history, and the like. Neither the investigators nor the subjects know who is getting the active drug and who is getting the placebo (hence, the term double-blind trial).

After the subjects are randomized, they then are followed to see how many in each group experience a *hard endpoint*. *(A hard endpoint is an event for which there are well-defined criteria, which might include specific symptoms or blood test results.)* In studies of heart disease, these are usually nonfatal heart attacks and death due to heart disease. Other endpoints sometimes are also analyzed; for example, the number of people experiencing strokes, or needing bypass surgery or angioplasties, and the total number of deaths.

The protocols for these trials must be approved by the institutional review board (IRB) of the hospital or clinic performing the study, and by the National Institutes of Health, if they are sponsoring the study. All of these trials also have a *data monitoring and safety board*, made up of experts who are not otherwise involved in the study. They meet on a regular basis, usually monthly, and they *do know* who is getting the real drug and who is getting placebo. If they find that one group is doing significantly better (or worse) than the other, the study is stopped prematurely and the results are published in a medical journal (and written about/discussed in the media).

There have been three primary prevention trials of statin drugs that have involved a total of 23,505 people. Each of these three trials showed that treating people who had no documented heart disease (but were at high risk of heart disease because of abnormal blood lipids or other risk factors) with a statin medicine lowered the risk of future cardiac events. Unfortunately, women made up only 12.5 percent of the people in these studies, and when their results were analyzed separately, there was no difference in the number of events that occurred in women whether they received a statin or placebo. (The numbers were 26 events in 1478 women on statin versus 30 events in 1461 women on placebo, a difference that was not significant. On the other hand, there were 190 events in 6992 men on statins versus 307 events in 6979 men on placebo, a difference that was highly significant.) The upshot of all this is that researcher know men without diagnosed vascular disease who are at high risk of developing ASCVD will lower that risk if they are treated with statins. Researchers cannot say this with any degree of assurance about women.

There have been many secondary prevention trials with statins, involving tens of thousands of people. These studies have looked at people with both stable ASCVD and people with unstable disease, so-called *acute coronary syndromes*. These studies have shown that people, both men and women, with documented ASCVD can lower their risk of developing future events by taking a statin medication.

By pooling the results of several primary and secondary trials and analyzing them (this is called a *meta-analysis*), investigators learned that the 30,817 people enrolled in these studies, treated for an average of 5.4 years, experienced an average 20 percent drop in total cholesterol, a 28 percent drop in LDL-C, a 13 percent drop in triglycerides, and a 5 percent increase in HDL-C. Compared to the people on placebo, those on statins had a 31 percent reduction in the relative risk of a major coronary event and a 21 percent reduction in the relative risk of dying.

In the last few years, the National Cholesterol Education Program (NCEP) has published guidelines to help doctors manage their patients' lipids. NCEP sets goals for what LDL-C, triglyceride, and HDL-C levels should be. We know that the more risk factors you have, the more likely you are to build up plaque in your arteries, so the NCEP guidelines instruct physicians to take into account five risk factors (other than LDL-C) to determine whether someone is at low, intermediate, or high risk. The other five risk factors are age (45 or older in men, 55 or older in women), smoking, high blood pressure, low HDL-C (less than 40 mg/dl in men and less than 50 mg/dl in women), and a family history of premature coronary heart disease (CHD) in a first-degree male relative younger than 55 or a first-degree female relative younger than 65.

If you have no or one risk factor, then your LDL-C goal is less than 160 mg/dl. If you have two or more risk factors, your LDL-C goal is less than 130 mg/dl— and if you have CHD or its equivalent (diabetes or vascular disease in the brain, extremities, or abdomen), then your LDL-C goal is less than 100 mg/dl. More recently, the NCEP has suggested that for people with ASCVD at particularly high risk, such as those with acute coronary syndromes or vascular disease and multiple risk factors, LDL-C should be reduced to 70 mg/dl or less. Depending on how high the LDL-C is before treatment, this goal may or may not be attainable.

Just because your physician has prescribed a statin to lower your LDL-C, it does mean that you can eat anything you want. As I tell my patients: "You can eat your way through any statin." It is very important that you consume a heart healthy diet, which is a *plant-based* diet. Meat should be treated as a condiment, not an entrée (and contrary to popular opinion, chicken *is* meat). Avoid animal (saturated) fats, palm oil, and coconut oil. Consume at least five to seven servings of vegetables and fruit every day. Olive oil (high in monounsaturated fats which raise the level of HDL-C) should be your main source of fat calories. Dairy products should be those made with skim or 1 percent milk. Eat whole grains and foods made with whole grains, like brown rice, whole wheat bread, and whole wheat pasta. Avoid white bread because white flour has been stripped of most of its nutrients and fiber, leaving empty calories.

You especially want to avoid partially hydrogenated vegetable oils (trans fats), which are unfortunately ubiquitous in most processed foods and a number of restaurant and fast foods. Trans fats both increase LDL-C and lower HDL-C, precisely what you don't want. (Be sure to read food labels because food companies can say a product has "0 trans fat" if it has less than 0.5 mg of trans fats per serving; if the food label says it has *any* partially hydrogenated vegetable oils, don't buy it because you want to keep *all* trans fats out of your diet.)

What was just described is the Mediterranean diet, eaten in many countries around the Mediterranean Sea 50 years ago, before they started to import high-saturated fat, nutritionally poor fast foods. The Mediterranean diet was shown in the Lyons Diet Heart Study to lower the risk of recurrent heart attacks in people with vascular disease when compared with the usual "prudent" diet, even without any lowering of LDL-C levels.

If, despite following a heart healthy diet your physician advises you that your LDL-C is still not at goal, he or she will most likely prescribe a statin medicine. The first statin to be approved by the FDA was lovastatin in 1987. Statins work by inhibiting a key enzyme involved in the manufacture of cholesterol by the body. This enzyme is called 3-hydroxy-3-methylglutaryl coenzyme A reductase, abbreviated HMG-CoA. Not only do statins interfere with the production of cholesterol, they also cause an increase in the number of LDL-C receptors in liver cells, which then remove more LDL-C from the blood. The effect of statins on blood lipid levels can be seen after about a week and is maximal about 4 to 6 weeks after starting therapy.

When I start someone on a statin, I mention that they may feel like they are coming down with the flu for a few days. They may feel a little queasy, a little achy, a bit fatigued, but if these symptoms occur, they tend to resolve in 3 or 4 days and are not signs of a serious side effect. Sometimes statins cause abnormalities in liver function tests. If this occurs and is mild, it often resolves without stopping the statin. If the liver enzyme test is more than three times the upper limit of normal, however, the statin should be stopped. Statins should be used with caution in people who consume large amounts of alcohol and should not be given to people with active liver disease.

Some people taking a statin medication will experience muscle pains, what doctors call *myalgia*. Sometimes this will resolve with lowering the dose or switching to another statin. There has been one study that suggested that the supplement coenzyme Q10 improved muscle pain in people on statins but this has not been confirmed by other studies. Your doctor may check a blood test, called CPK, to see if there is any evidence of actual muscle damage, if you are experiencing muscle aches.

The most feared side effect of statin therapy is *rhabdomyolysis*. This rare condition is characterized by severe damage to skeletal muscles throughout the body, often accompanied by marked pain, weakness, dark urine, and in rare instances, kidney failure and death. The risk of rhabdomyolysis is increased if statins are given with certain other medicines, including some antibiotics, antifungal medicines, medicines used to treat HIV, verapamil, gemfibrozil, and drugs used to suppress the immune response in people who have had transplants. It is critical (and not just in the case of statins) that every doctor knows the name of every medicine you are taking, including over-the-counter medicines to lessen the chance of a dangerous drug interaction. The risk of rhabdomyolysis also is increased in the elderly, women, those with kidney disease, those with uncontrolled infections or seizures, and those taking high doses of statins.

Doubling the dose of a statin medicine causes an additional drop in LDL-C levels of about 6 percent, while increasing the risk of side effects. For this reason, if your LDL-C is not at goal, your doctor may either add a medicine that works by a different mechanism or prescribe one of the statin combination pills that are available.

If you have high levels of triglycerides, or low levels of HDL cholesterol after your elevated LDL cholesterol has been treated, your physician may add either a fibrate medicine or niacin to lower the residual risk of having a cardiovascular event that persists even after LDL cholesterol levels are brought down significantly.

While taking a statin, it is important that you notify your doctor if you develop **unusual** muscle pain, especially if it is diffuse, and associated with weakness, tenderness, and fever.

Cholesterol is essential for normal growth of a fetus. For this reason, statins should be avoided in women of childbearing age unless they are highly unlikely to conceive and have been informed of the danger should they become pregnant.

Statins, with the exception of atorvastatin and rosuvastatin, usually are taken at bedtime or with the evening meal. Of the statins, pravastatin and fluvastatin appear to be the least likely to interact with other medications, due to the way their metabolism is handled by the liver.

Again, it is crucial that all your doctors know **all** the medicines you are taking before they prescribe anything new.

Table 1–19 lists the statins currently available in the United States, along with two combination pills.

Table 1–19 Statins

Drug (Trade) Name	Dosage Range (mg/dl)
Atorvastatin (Lipitor®)	10–80
Fluvastatin (Lescol®)	20–80
Lovastatin (Mevacor®)	10–80
Pravastatin (Pravachol®)	10–80
Rosuvastatin (Crestor®)	5–40
Simvastatin (Zocor®)	10–80

Statin Combinations

Drug (Trade) Name	Dosage Range (mg/dl)
Lovastatin/niacin (Advicor®)	500/20–2,000/40
Simvastatin/ezetimibe (Vytorin®)	10/10–80/10

Fibrates

The first of the fibrate drugs, clofibrate, was discovered in the early 1960s. Shortly thereafter, clofibrate was one of the medicines used in an early secondary prevention trial, the Coronary Drug Project, which took place between 1966 and 1975. This study enrolled over 8000 men who had survived a heart attack and randomized them to five treatment arms and one placebo arm. The aim was to see if lowering cholesterol would lower the risk of future cardiac events in these men. The five treatment arms utilized either a low or a high dose of estrogen, niacin, thyroid hormone, or clofibrate. The high-dose estrogen arm was stopped early because these men were having more heart attacks and deaths than the men getting the placebo. The lose-dose estrogen arm was stopped a few years later because men on low-dose estrogen were doing no better than the men on placebo, but were having an unacceptable side effect: enlargement of the breasts. (While many men seem to like large breasts in women, growing a set of their own was clearly unacceptable.) By the time the trial ended, there was no evidence of a reduction in risk in the clofibrate group or the group receiving thyroid hormone (this arm also was stopped prematurely because of side effects). The group treated with niacin had a reduction in their risk of recurrent heart attack, but no decrease in their risk of dying. Of interest, nine years after the end of the trial, the death rate from all causes was similar in all the groups except for the group of men who had taken niacin, in whom mortality was reduced by 11 percent. It is unclear to what caused this late benefit, occurring after the niacin was discontinued.

This early negative study did not prevent researchers from looking for other drugs of the fibrate class that might be more beneficial. In the 1980s, a study in Finland, the Helsinki Heart Study, found that another fibrate, gemfibrozil, lowered the risk of cardiac events in a primary prevention trial of over 4000 men who had elevations of triglycerides and low HDL-C. A secondary prevention trial in the United States that used gemfibrozil also had a positive result. More recently, a large trial in people with diabetes showed a benefit in reducing the risk of total cardiovascular events (nonfatal heart attack, stroke, cardiac death, and cardiac or carotid artery revascularization) in people treated with the newest fibrate, fenofibrate.

There have been no studies showing a beneficial effect of clofibrate in lowering the risk for cardiac events, and one study showed that it lead to an increase in abnormal heart rhythms. For this reason, it rarely is used today, except to treat a rare lipid disorder called *Type III hyperlipoproteinemia*, a familial disease in which there is an increased risk of premature vascular disease.

Fibrates work by decreasing the production of very low density lipoprotein cholesterol (VLDL-C) and increasing its clearance from the bloodstream. They also increase HDL-C production. People treated with fibrates have a decrease in their triglycerides levels and an increase in their HDL-C levels. Although the older fibrates had little effect on LDL-C levels, treatment with fenofibrate may lead

Table 1–20 Fibrates

Drug (Trade) Name	Dosage Range (mg/dl)
Clofibrate (Atromid-S®)	2,000
Fenofibrate (Tricor®)	48–145
Gemfibrozil (Lopid®)	1,200

to modest reductions in LDL-C. In addition, it makes LDL particles larger and more buoyant, which is felt to make them less likely to cause plaques. Fenofibrate, like niacin and unlike statins, also lowers level of Lp(a).

Fibrates have been associated with an increased risk of gallstones. In addition, they may cause bloating and nausea, abnormal liver function tests, and may increase the effect of the blood thinner warfarin. If you are on warfarin or Coumadin® and you start a fibrate, your dose of the blood thinner should be reduced and you should have frequent blood tests until your proper dose has been determined. Rarely, like statins, rhabdomyolysis has occurred in people treated with fibrates. Gemfibrozil, but not fenofibrate, when used with a statin, causes the blood level of the statin to be increased. This is a possible reason why the risk of rhabdomyolysis is higher with the combination of statin and gemfibrozil than statin and fenofibrate. Gemfibrozil and clofibrate are taken twice a day, 30 minutes before meals. Fenofibrate is taken once a day.

Table 1–20 lists the fibrates that are currently available in the United States.

Ezetimibe

Ezetimibe is the newest cholesterol-lowering medicine to be approved by the FDA and it works in a way that is different from all of the others: It doesn't interfere with the liver's production of lipoproteins nor does it bind to bile acids. Instead, it works by blocking the absorption of cholesterol from the small intestine, which is derived from two sources: the food we eat, but in much larger amounts, the cholesterol secreted in the bile. Ezetimibe blocks the absorption of cholesterol from both these sources leading to a reduction in total cholesterol, triglycerides, and LDL-C. There usually is no change or a slight increase in HDL-C. When used alone in people with high cholesterol, ezetimibe causes LDL-C levels to drop by about 18 percent, and triglyceride level to drop by about 8 percent. Most often, however, ezetimibe is given in conjunction with another type of lipid-lowering medicine, such as a statin or a fibrate. In studies comparing ezetimibe alone with placebo, there was no difference in the likelihood of developing abnormal liver function tests in people taking ezetimibe. Ezetimibe does not appear to cause the muscle damage that can occur in people taking statins or fibrates.

Ezetimibe is given once a day and can be taken without regard to meals. Unlike bile acid sequestrants, ezetimibe is absorbed into the body. There are no scientific studies of ezetimibe in pregnant women and its use in pregnancy or in nursing mothers is not recommended unless the potential benefit outweighs the risk.

In early 2008, the results of the ENHANCE trial became available. This study compared ezetimibe plus simvastatin to placebo plus simvastatin in 720 people with familial hypercholesterolemia. They had severe elevations of LDL-C averaging 319 mg/dl. There was no statistically significant difference in IMT between the two groups, despite the fact that those treated with ezetimibe/simvastatin had an average reduction in LDL-C of 58 percent compared to an average reduction of 41 percent in those treated with simvastatin/placebo. There was a tendency for carotid IMT to increase in those treated with ezetimibe/simvastatin compared to simvastatin/placebo, but this difference did not achieve statistical "significance", that is it might have occurred by chance alone.

ENHANCE was the type of study called a "surrogate end-point" trial, that is, rather than looking at "hard" end-points such as heart attack, stroke or death, the researchers measured something called *carotid intima-media thickness* (IMT) using ultrasound waves. IMT is felt to be a "surrogate" for clinical events, but looking at surrogate end-points may be misleading. For example, a study published in the American Journal of Epidemiology in 1994 looked at carotid IMT measured by ultrasound in post-menopausal women and concluded that those taking estrogen-replacement therapy (ERT) had a decrease in carotid IMT and women who were not taking ERT had an increase in carotid IMT. However, in subsequent studies which looked at hard end-points, postmenopausal women who took hormone replacement therapy, whether estrogen alone or a combination of estrogen and progesterone actually had a significant increase in strokes compared to women on placebo.

The definitive end-point trials to determine if adding ezetimibe to a statin further reduces the risk of heart attack, stroke and death compared to therapy with statin alone are underway. There are three such trials involving more than 20,000 subjects and their results are expected by 2011.

Fatigue and diarrhea seem to be the most frequent side effects occurring in about 2 to 4 percent of people. Allergic reactions also can occur, usually in the form of a rash.

Table 1–21 lists ezetimibe and a statin/ezetimide combination available in the United States.

Table 1–21 Available Ezetimibe and a Statin/Ezetimide Combination

Drug (Trade) Name	Dosage Range (mg/d)
Ezetimibe (Zetia®)	10
Ezetimibe/simvastatin (Vytorin®)	10/10–10/80

Omega-3 Fatty Acids

For many years, fats have had a bad reputation, mainly because Americans consume far too many of them and often choose the most unhealthy forms, saturated and trans fats. A little background information about fats will help clear up some of the confusion many people have on this subject.

Fats are chemical compounds made up of *glycerol* (also called *glycerine*) bound to fatty acids. Glycerol is composed of carbon, hydrogen, and oxygen; tastes sweet; and can be dissolved in water. Fatty acids also are composed of carbon, hydrogen, and oxygen. They contain anywhere from 4 to 24 carbon atoms per molecule and varying amounts of hydrogen. The terms *saturated, monounsaturated,* and *polyunsaturated* refer to the number of double bonds the fat molecule contains. A double bond occurs when two atoms are bound by two pairs of electrons rather than one. If the carbon in a fatty acid has all the hydrogen it can hold, it is called a saturated fat and will not have any double bonds between carbon and hydrogen. Monounsaturated fats have one double bond and polyunsaturated fats have two or more double bonds. In the following illustration, H stands for hydrogen, C stands for carbon, and O stands for oxygen. There is a double bond between the carbon and oxygen but not between any carbon and hydrogen atom.

This simple fat, butyric acid, is therefore a saturated fat. The carbon atom on the right side of the molecule is attached to two oxygen atoms and a hydrogen atom. This is called a *carboxyl group* and this end of the molecule is called the *alpha end.* The other end is called the *omega end.* To simplify a complex subject, saturated fats raise the level of LDL-C and are bad for us. Monounsaturated fats raise the level of HDL-C and are good for us. Polyunsaturated fats come in many forms but the two most important are called *omega-3* and *omega-6*.

Omega-3 and omega-6 fatty acids are polyunsaturated fats that have a double bond either three or six carbons from the omega end. They are called *essential fatty acids* because the body cannot make them so they must be consumed in the diet. The omega-3 fatty acids appear to have many health benefits. The evidence for benefit in lowering the risk of heart disease is best for omega-3 fatty acids derived

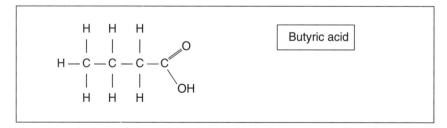

Figure 1–1 Fatty Acid

from fatty fish, such as salmon, trout, and herring. These fish contain significant amounts of *eicosapentaenoic acid* (*EPA*) and *docosahexaenoic acid* (*DHA*). In studies of countries where people consume large amounts of fish, there appears to be a lower risk of sudden cardiac death than in countries like the United States where fish consumption is much less. In one RCT of survivors of heart attack, men randomized to fish oil supplements had a 25 percent lower risk of a subsequent cardiac event compared to men taking a placebo.

Large doses of omega-3 fatty acids lower levels of triglyceride. Omega-3 fatty acids also have antioxidant and anti-inflammatory effects. On the other hand, there is some evidence that the intake of excessive amounts of omega-6 fatty acids is associated with chronic diseases including some forms of cancer, heart disease, and arthritis. There are countless omega-3 supplements on the market. These are derived from either fish or plant sources (walnuts, flax seed, and canola oil are rich in omega-3s). Like all supplements, they are not subject to the same oversight by the FDA that prescription medicines are and for this reason there is legitimate cause for concern about safety and purity, particularly of fish oil supplements.

The American Heart Association currently recommends that people with documented coronary heart disease eat about one gram of EPA and DHA a day, preferably in the form of fatty fish. This dose, however, is not sufficient to lower elevated triglyceride levels. Three to 4 grams of omega-3 fatty acids are needed to treat high levels of triglyceride.

Currently, the only FDA-approved prescription omega-3 fatty acid supplement is Lovaza. It is indicated to treat people who have very high fasting triglyceride values of 500 mg/dl or more. Lovaza is highly purified and therefore does not carry a risk of mercury or PCB contamination. In addition, it contains more DHA/EPA (84 percent) than unregulated supplements which may contain anywhere from 13 to 63 percent DHA/EPA.

In 1956, hundreds of people died from eating mercury-contaminated fish from Minamata Bay in Japan. Thousands of others were left with permanent brain damage. Since that time, mercury contamination of fish from all over the globe has been documented. Mercury concentrations tends to be higher in the large fish at the top of the food chain, such as tuna, king mackerel, and swordfish and for this reason, pregnant women and children are advised to avoid eating these fish.

In addition, polychlorinated biphenyls (PCBs) are industrial pollutants that have been found in fish, especially some farmed fish. PCBs have been found to be cancer causing in animals, and when humans suffer PCB exposure, the effects include acne-like skin rashes, behavioral changes, and interference with the immune system. Although only small amounts of mercury and PCBs have been found in over-the-counter fish oil supplements, the problem with these products lies in the fact that they are not subject to regulation by the FDA and could have higher levels than are safe, depending on the origin of the fish used in their manufacture.

The usual dose is four 1-gram capsules taken once daily or two 1-gram capsules twice daily. The most frequently reported side effects include belching, flu-like symptoms, dyspepsia, fishy aftertaste, back pain, and rash. Some studies of omega-3 fatty acids have shown prolongation of a test called *bleeding time*. However, the increase was not enough to make the bleeding time abnormal and did not seem to lead to an increased risk of bleeding.

Lovaza reduces triglycerides by about 45 percent and raises HDL-C about 9 percent. People with very high triglycerides who are treated with Omacor have been noted to have increases in their LDL-C. However, lowering triglycerides causes LDL-C to become less dense, and in this form, LDL-C is considered to be less likely to cause plaque formation.

People with fish allergy should not take Lovaza and because its use in pregnant women has not been studied, it should be prescribed during pregnancy only if the potential benefits outweigh the potential risk. Table 1–22 lists the FDA-approved prescription omega-3 supplement available in the United States.

Table 1–22 Omega-3 Fatty Acid

Drug (Trade) Name	Dosage Range (g/d)
Omega-3 fatty acid (Lovaza®)	3–4

MEDICINES TO TREAT NICOTINE ADDICTION

The smoking or chewing of tobacco was unknown to the western world until Columbus' voyages of discovery in 1492. He wrote about highly prized dried leaves that were given to him as a gift by the Arawaks on the island he dubbed San Salvador. (He promptly threw them away.) This was the first known instance of tobacco being offered to a European. Impressed by how popular they were with the natives, on subsequent trips Columbus brought tobacco leaves back to Spain and it wasn't long before tobacco use was widespread throughout Europe.

Tobacco had been cultivated throughout North, South, and Central America for thousands of years. It was smoked or chewed and played a role in the religious ceremonies of many tribes. Although the origin of the practice is unknown, tobacco enemas for a time were all the rage in 18th century Europe. Less than one hundred years after Columbus' first voyage to the Americas, a Spanish physician, Nicolas Monardes, in a book about medicinal plants of the New World, claimed that tobacco cured 36 diseases! (This was before the era of randomized controlled trials.)

The tobacco plant was given the name *Nicotiana tabacum* in honor of Jean Nicot, a 16th-century French scholar and diplomat who brought it from Portugal to France and wrote about its medicinal uses. His name also is immortalized in the word *nicotine*, the highly addictive active substance in tobacco. Nicot brought tobacco to the attention of the French queen, Catherine de Medici, who was so impressed with its effect on her migraine headaches that she decreed it should be called "Herba Regina," the queen's herb. Nicotine is a powerful poison. (Ironically, Catherine de Medici has a perhaps well-deserved reputation as a successful poisoner.) Just one cigarette contains enough nicotine to kill an average 3-year-old were he or she to eat it. Over time, the early enthusiasm for nicotine gradually gave way to increasing recognition of its many harmful effects.

The addictive potential of nicotine is well known to smokers. Nicotine is estimated to be three to ten times more addicting than heroin. In addition to nicotine, there are more than 4000 other chemicals found in cigarettes and their smoke, including 69 that are *carcinogenic*; that is, they lead to the development of cancer. These other chemicals include carbon monoxide, benzene, toluene, hydrogen cyanide, formaldehyde, ammonia, and polonium-210 (the notorious isotope that caused the fatal poisoning of the Russian dissident, Alexander Litvinenko).

Studies in the 1950s showed unequivocally that smoking cigarettes caused lung cancer. At about the same time, as a result of the Framingham Study, cigarette smoking was shown to be a powerful risk factor for the development of atherosclerotic cardiovascular disease. In fact, cigarette smoking is the number one cause of preventable premature death in this country. An estimated 440,000 people die in the United States each year from smoking-related diseases, chiefly cardiovascular. Worldwide, cigarette smoking is responsible for about 5 million deaths annually.

Smoking increases the risk of ASCVD by several mechanisms. It lowers the level of HDL-C. The carbon monoxide and many of the other chemicals in smoke directly injure the walls of arteries, and anything that injures arteries increases plaque formation. Smoking increases pulse and blood pressure, increasing the work of the heart. It makes the blood more likely to clot, and when clots form in the arteries of the heart, the result is often a heart attack. When clotting occurs in the arteries in the brain, the result is often a stroke. Smoking even increases the risk of developing diabetes. Women who smoke two or more packs of cigarettes a day increase their risk of developing diabetes by 74 percent. Men who smoke two or more packs of cigarettes a day increase their risk of diabetes by 45 percent. Women who smoke, on average, experience menopause 1.5 to 2 years earlier than nonsmokers. One study found that smoking lowered the median age of first heart attack by 19 years in women and 7 years in men. Aneurysms (ballooning and weakening of an artery) of the abdominal aorta occur many times more often in smokers than nonsmokers.

Smoking increases the risk of not only lung cancer but also head, mouth, throat, bladder, pancreatic, cervical, esophageal, and kidney cancer. It causes erectile dysfunction, blockages in leg arteries leading to gangrene, gum disease, bad breath, and premature wrinkling and aging of the skin. Women who smoke during pregnancy have a higher rate of obstetric complications and lower birth-weight babies. Were nicotine not so powerfully addictive, no one in their right mind would smoke! I tell my patients that smoking is just a socially acceptable form of suicide, and that the tobacco industry is the most successful organized crime syndicate in the country (and the world). It kills more people than any other crime syndicate; it makes more money than any other crime syndicate—and for reasons that are murky at best and shameful at worst, the manufacture and sale of cigarettes is perfectly legal!

The first pharmacologic method to help smokers quit involved prescribing nicotine gum. For the last several years, nicotine gum, patches, and lozenges have been available without a prescription. They all decrease the withdrawal symptoms that occur when a nicotine-addicted person stops smoking. However, studies have shown that people are much more likely to be successful quitters if, in addition to using nicotine replacement products, they attend a stop-smoking program. Most hospitals have such programs, which cost a nominal amount, but far less than the average smoker spends on cigarettes.

The next section will discuss the prescription drugs that are available to help smokers beat nicotine addiction.

Bupropion

Bupropion is an antidepressant which, in 1997, won FDA approval for treating nicotine addiction. Smokers begin taking bupropion in a sustained release form 1 week before their quit date. They start by taking one pill containing 150 mg/day for 3 days, then increase the dose to 150 mg twice a day. The two doses should be taken at least 8 hours apart. The pills need to be swallowed whole, not chewed, crushed, or cut in half. Bupropion lessens the craving for nicotine by an unknown mechanism. Treatment usually is continued for 7 to 8 weeks. If someone has been unsuccessful in stopping after 8 weeks, bupropion is unlikely to work and the medicine is stopped.

Allergic reactions, in the form of rash, or itching swelling around the face and mouth, can occur, but are rare. Occasionally hypertension can occur, especially if bupropion is taken with a nicotine replacement gum or patch. The most serious potential side effect is a seizure, and bupropion should not be prescribed to people who have epilepsy or a seizure disorder, to people who drink alcohol to excess, or to people who abuse other drugs. As with other antidepressants, there is a risk of suicidal thoughts and suicide in people with major depression treated with bupropion. Its safety in pregnancy is not known but because it is excreted in milk, nursing mothers should not receive bupropion.

Table 1–23 Nicotine Addiction Drugs

Drug (Trade) Name	Usual dose (mg/day)
Bupropion (Zyban®, Wellbutrin SR®, Wellbutrin XL®)	300
Varenicline (Chantix®)	1.0–2.0

Varenicline

The latest drug approved by the FDA to treat nicotine addiction and help smokers to quit is varenicline. Like bupropion, varenicline works on the brain to reduce symptoms of nicotine withdrawal. In addition, it blocks some of the pleasurable effects of nicotine in people who resume smoking while taking varenicline. In most of the clinical trials that proved its usefulness, varenicline, like bupropion was begun a week prior to a quit date. In a head-to-head study between varenicline and bupropion, more people remained smoke-free with the former at 9 to 12 weeks, but at the end of 52 weeks, there was no difference in the percentage of people remaining smoke-free on either drug. Unlike bupropion, there does not seem to be any risk of seizures in people treated with varenicline.

Like bupropion, varenicline is taken by mouth twice a day. The most common side effects of varenicline are nausea, vomiting, insomnia, gas, headache, bad dreams, and alteration in taste. Varenicline is taken after meals with water. The dose is increased gradually from 0.5 mg once a day for the first 3 days, to 0.5 mg twice daily on days 4 thru 7, to 1.0 mg twice daily from day 8 until the end of treatment (usually 12 weeks). If the treatment is not successful at 12 weeks, varenicline is stopped. However, in people who quit successfully, an additional 12 weeks of therapy is recommended to increase the chance of long-term quitting. This medicine should not be taken by people under the age of 18, or by pregnant or nursing women since the safety of varenicline in these groups has not been tested. Table 1–23 lists the prescription medicines used to help smokers quit.

CHAPTER 2

Treating Angina Pectoris

In 1768, a well-known British physician by the name of William Heberden gave an address to the Royal College of Physicians in London. Like all learned men of his time, he spoke and wrote in Latin. He described a new syndrome to which he gave the name *angina pectoris*.

His speech was published 4 years later in the *Transactions of the Royal College* and is excerpted here:

> But there is a disorder of the breast marked with strong and peculiar symptoms, considerable for the kind of danger belonging to it, and not extremely rare, which deserves to be mentioned more at length. The seat of it, and sense of strangling, and anxiety with which it is attended, may make it not improperly be called angina pectoris.
>
> They who are afflicted with it, are seized while they are walking, (more especially if it be up hill, and soon after eating) with a painful and most disagreeable sensation in the breast, which seems as if it would extinguish life, if it were to increase or continue; but the moment they stand still, all this uneasiness vanishes . . . .
>
> Males are most liable to that disease, especially such as have passed their fiftieth year . . . . I have seen nearly a hundred people under this disorder, of which number there have been three women . . . . The termination of the angina pectoris is remarkable. For, if no accidents intervene, but the disease goes on to its height, the patients all suddenly fall down, and perish almost immediately. *Commentaries on the history and cure of diseases.* (Heberden, William, 1710–1801, New York, published under the auspices of The Library of New York Academy of Medicine by Hafner Publishing Co., 1962.)

This was the first description of angina to appear in the medical literature. Although Heberden gave an excellent description of this symptom, he thought it was due to a cramp or an ulcer. Because the pulse was usually normal during an attack, he discounted the possibility that angina was caused by some cardiac condition. It was Heberden's friend Edward Jenner who first suggested, in 1786, that angina pectoris was caused by "ossification" (calcification, or, in other words, hardening) of the coronary arteries after observing an autopsy on a man who had suffered from angina. (Today, Jenner is remembered as the physician who first proved that a vaccine made from cowpox pus would prevent smallpox.) Jenner wrote a letter to Heberden in which he noted "the importance of the coronary arteries, and how

much the heart must suffer from their not being able to perform their functions .
. . ." Then in 1799, another British physician, Caleb Parry wrote a monograph en-
titled *An Inquiry into the Symptoms and Causes of Syncope Anginosa, Commonly
Called Angina Pectoris* in which he credited Edward Jenner with the theory that
angina was caused by disease in the coronary arteries. Parry was the first person
to suggest ways of preventing coronary artery disease. To this end, he advocated
moderation in eating and drinking, the avoidance of "flesh meats," and "moderate
bodily exercise," instructions that are echoed by doctors in the 21st century. We
now know that angina is caused by *ischemia*, a relative lack of blood supply to the
heart muscle, which occurs in people with a buildup of plaque in the arteries to the
heart.

It was not until a half a century later that effective treatments for angina pectoris
were discovered. The first of these was a compound called *amyl nitrite*, which was
synthesized by a French chemist, Antoine Balard, in 1844.

Meanwhile, in 1846, an Italian physician by the name of Ascanio Sobrero discovered another compound, glyceryl trinitrate, which he called *nitroglycerin*. His
face was later scarred from a laboratory accident in which the nitroglycerin he was
working with exploded. Alfred Nobel, who made provisions in his will for the prize
that was named after him, worked in the same laboratory as Sobrero, and went on
to invent dynamite and a blasting cap, which reduced the dangers of working with
nitroglycerin. Ironically, later in life when Nobel, by then a very wealthy man, developed angina himself and was prescribed nitroglycerin, he refused to take it.

In the 1860s, a Scottish physician by the name of T. Lauder Brunton studied the
effect of amyl nitrite on patients in the Edinburgh Royal Infirmary. He found that
if he gave it to patients with angina, their discomfort would almost always resolve
in under a minute. Brunton published his observations in the British journal *Lancet*
in1867. He went on to study nitroglycerin but never suggested it be used to treat
angina; he stopped work with it because it gave him severe headaches.

The first physician to demonstrate the effectiveness of nitroglycerin in the treatment of angina was William Murrell. He wrote a long article in *Lancet* in 1879,
"Nitro-glycerine as a Remedy for Angina Pectoris," in which he detailed the results
of experiments he performed on himself and on patients. He noted that the effects
of nitroglycerin lasted some 30 minutes, whereas with amyl nitrite, effects were
dissipated within about 90 seconds. To this day, nitroglycerin is the mainstay of
treatment for the symptom of angina pectoris. Along with digitalis, it is the only
part of the cardiac medical armamentarium that has been in use for more than a
century. The vast majority of other cardiac medicines have been in use for under
30 years. (In fact, most of the medicines I prescribe every day were not available
when I graduated from medical school in 1968.)

Nitroglycerin and the other nitrate medicines work by dilating blood vessels,
both veins and arteries. They also are used in the treatment of congestive heart failure, a condition in which the heart is incapable of pumping enough blood for the
body's needs. When atherosclerosis narrows an artery supplying the heart muscle
(there are two of these so-called "coronary" arteries), an adequate supply of blood

flow to the heart may be supplied when the body is at rest. However, when the demands on the heart are increased, with exercise or emotional stress, not enough blood may get by the narrowing (also called a *stenosis*) to provide the heart muscle with the increased blood it needs, inducing the condition called *ischemia* and usually, the symptom we call angina.

Nitroglycerin dilates not only the blood vessels in the heart, but all the blood vessels throughout the body. Sometimes this causes a pounding headache. I tell my patients: "That's a good sign. It's a sign that it's working." Nitroglycerin pills lose potency over time, especially when exposed to air, so they should be kept tightly capped in the little bottle they come in and discarded 6 months after opening. Nitroglycerin also usually causes a bit of burning under the tongue, so if you notice that this is no longer the case, it's time to replace your nitroglycerin tablets. The other not uncommon side effect is a drop in blood pressure. I always instruct my patients to sit down before the first time they take nitroglycerin; then if their blood pressure drops and they get dizzy, they are less likely to fall or pass out. If despite sitting they still feel dizzy, I tell them to lie down and elevate their legs. This is almost always sufficient to bring the blood pressure back up and prevent a fainting spell. The side effect of a drop in blood pressure is more apt to occur if one is dehydrated so people on nitrates need to be careful to drink adequate amounts of fluid.

There are also other medicines that increase the likelihood of a drop in blood pressure in people on nitrates. The most dangerous interaction occurs if one of the medicines to treat erectile dysfunction is taken within 24 hours of nitroglycerin or other nitrate medicine. Viagra®, Levitra®, and Cialis® should not be taken within 24 hours of any nitrate. Doing so may cause a dangerous drop in blood pressure, which could result in fainting or a heart attack. People taking other vasodilators, such as those used to treat high blood pressure, also are more likely to experience a drop in their blood pressure when taking nitroglycerin.

Nitroglycerin may be taken to end an attack of angina or to prevent one. Its onset of action is within minutes of placing a pill under the tongue. When taken to prevent an angina attack, we call this *prophylactic nitroglycerin*. For example, if a patient knows that every time she climbs the cellar stairs carrying a load of laundry she develops angina, she can take a nitroglycerin ahead of time and prevent it.

It is important that people take nitroglycerin as soon as they experience angina. While the heart is ischemic, it is starved for oxygen, and more prone to abnormal heart rhythms. It also can't beat as strongly as it should, and the resting pressure inside the heart becomes elevated, often causing shortness of breath. If the attack of angina is not relieved in 5 minutes, another dose of nitroglycerin is taken. After another 5 minutes without relief, another nitroglycerin dose can be taken but if that doesn't lead to relief in 5 minutes, it's time to call the emergency squad and get to the nearest emergency room.

I tell my patients that even if they're not sure that what they are feeling is angina, if it's not their heart, nitroglycerin won't hurt. If it is their heart, nitroglycerin will help—and it's far better to go the emergency room only find out that you're having a gall bladder attack than to stay at home, have a heart attack, and perhaps die. Women seem to have a particularly hard time thinking it might be their heart when they have chest discomfort. Studies have shown that they delay seeking medical attention longer than men in that situation and this might partially account for the fact that a woman is more apt to die when she has a heart attack than a man is.

Nitroglycerin comes in pill form and as a spray. The pill is placed under the tongue where it dissolves. This allows for rapid uptake of nitroglycerin into the bloodstream. Likewise, nitroglycerin spray is directed under the tongue. Both the pills and the spray are short-acting nitrates, with the effect lasting for about 30 minutes. There now are longer acting nitrates, which can be taken either as pills or through the skin in the form of patches or paste. Nitroglycerin patches release a constant amount of nitroglycerin into the blood and are usually worn for 12 hours a day. Nitroglycerin paste is measured out and smeared onto the skin until it's a thin transparent film and then covered with plastic wrap to prevent it getting on clothes. Nitroglycerin paste usually is applied two or three times a day.

People who have taken nitrates for many years may build up a tolerance. When this happens they may require increased doses to get the same amount of relief. Table 2–1 lists some of the available nitroglycerin preparations and their dosages.

There are long-acting nitrate preparations that are chemically different from nitroglycerine. These long-acting nitrates are used prophylactically to prevent angina, not to treat acute attacks because they are not absorbed quickly enough to treat angina acutely. Like short-acting nitroglycerin, they may cause headache, but they are less likely to cause dizziness and a marked drop in blood pressure. The most commonly prescribed long-acting nitrate is called *isosorbide*. The long-acting preparations are meant to be swallowed. Be sure you understand the proper way to take your prescription because the extended release form of isosorbide should not be crushed or chewed.

Table 2–2 lists some of the commonly prescribed long-acting oral nitrates and their usual daily dosages. Some of these medicines are taken once a day, others are taken two or three times a day. Your physician will tell you how many times a day you need to take your long-acting nitrate. Just as with nitroglycerine, tolerance to

Table 2–1 Nitrates

Drug (Trade)Name	Dosage Range (mg)
Nitroglycerin (Nitrostat®, Nitro-Dur®, Nitrogard®)	0.2–0.6
Nitroglycerin Spray (Nitrolingual®)	0.4 per squirt
Nitroglycerin Paste (Minitran®, Transderm Nitro®)	0.5–1.0 inch 2 or 3 times/d
Nitroglycerin Patch (Nitro-Dur patch®, Minitran Patch®)	0.2–0.8 mg/hour for 12 hours

Table 2–2 Long Acting Oral Nitrates

Drug (Trade) Name	Dosage Range mg/d
Isosorbide dinitrate (Isordil®, Sorbitrate®, Dilatrate-SR®)	15–120
Isosorbide-5-mononitrate (Imdur®, Ismo®)	30–120

isosorbide can develop and lead to a need for increased dosages. Tolerance often can be avoided by ensuring a 14-hour nitrate-free interval each day.

BETA-BLOCKERS

We've already discussed the use of beta-blockers in the treatment of high blood pressure, but they are even more of a mainstay in the treatment of angina. In fact, unless there is some very strong reason why beta-blockers should not be used (what is called a *contraindication*), every patient who suffers from angina should be treated with a beta-blocker. Some of the reasons why this class of medicine might be contraindicated include severe asthma, uncontrolled heart failure, or severe slowing of the heart rate as is seen in various forms of *heart block*.

The heart is a four-chambered muscular pump. There are two receiving chambers called the *right atrium* and *left atrium* and two pumping chambers called the *right ventricle* and the *left ventricle*. The right side of the heart receives venous blood that has given up oxygen and nutrients to the cells and pumps it via the pulmonary artery into the lungs where it takes in oxygen and gives up carbon dioxide. The left side of the heart takes the oxygenated blood from the lungs and pumps it via the aorta all over the body. (The network of blood vessels that supplies the body's organs is called the *systemic circulation*; the network of blood vessels that goes to the lung is called the *pulmonary circulation*.) Like all pumps, the heart needs energy. It gets its energy from the oxygen in the blood and it gets its own blood supply from the right and left coronary arteries, which are the very first branches given off by the aorta, the artery that carries arterial blood from the left ventricle. Figure 2–1 shows you this anatomy.

Several factors determine how much oxygen the heart muscle needs at any point in time. Three of the most important are the heart rate (the number of times the heart contracts in a minute), the amount of pressure the heart has to contract against (called the *impedance*; it correlates roughly with the systolic blood pressure) and contractility (the rate at which the heart develops pressure when it contracts). Beta-blockers blunt the increase in pulse, blood pressure, and contractility that occurs with exercise or stress and prevents the heart from becoming *ischemic* (relatively lacking in blood supply) when it needs more oxygen but the blood flow to the heart muscle is compromised by an atherosclerotic narrowing in a coronary artery.

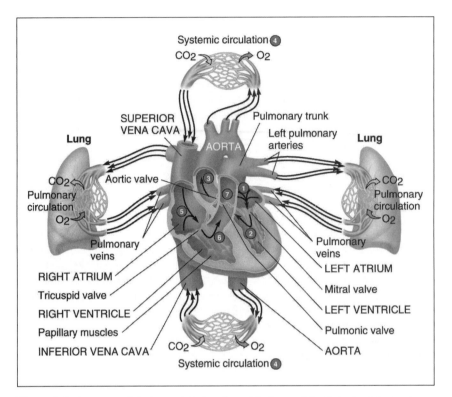

Figure 2–1 Anatomy of the heart: 1 Left atrium. 2 Left ventricle. 3 Aorta. 4 Systemic circulation. 5 Right atrium. 6 Right ventricle. 7 Pulmonary artery.

Courtesy of Jones & Bartlett

When the heart is ischemic, it is more prone to abnormal heart rhythms *(arrhythmias)*, which could be fatal. Beta-blockers also decrease the risk of arrhythmias, both when the heart is ischemic and even when it is not. All in all, beta-blockers are extremely safe and effective medicines in people with coronary artery disease.

Table 2–3 lists the beta-blockers that are approved to treat angina. For a discussion of possible side effects, refer to the discussion in the beta-blockers' section of Chapter 1, which precedes these tables. It should be noted that the newest beta-blocker to be approved by the FDA, nevibolol has been approved to treat hypertension only. In addition, people who have angina may experience an increase in attacks, if they discontinue beta-blockers abruptly. People with angina should, if at all possible, taper the dose of beta-blocker under their physician's direction of a beta-blocker needs to be discontinued.

Table 2–3 Beta-blockers for treating angina

Drug (Trade) Name	Usual Dose mg/d
Atenolol (Tenormin®)	25–100
Metoprolol (Lopressor®, Toprol®, Toprol XL®)	25–200
Nadolol (Corgard®)	40–320
Propranolol (Inderal®, Inderal LA®)	40–240

Calcium Channel Blockers

CCBs can be added to nitrates and beta-blockers to treat angina or they may be used instead of beta-blockers in people who have a contraindication to the latter. The nondihydropyridine CCBs decrease the heart rate and contractility, decreasing the heart's need for oxygen, in addition to relaxing the smooth muscle in the coronary arteries, thereby allowing them to dilate. For this reason, they should not be used in people with significant congestive heart failure or very slow heart rates. The dihydropyridine CCBs don't affect the heart rate or contractility so they *can* be used in people with very slow heart rates or congestive heart failure. For further information, please refer back to tables 1–11 and 1–12.

RANOLAZINE

In January 2006, the FDA approved a new medicine for the treatment of angina. Ranolazine does not work by relaxing blood vessels or decreasing pulse or blood pressure. In fact, researchers are not sure why it is effective in lowering the frequency of angina attacks, but it appears to work at the level of the cardiac muscle cell to improve the efficiency of oxygen utilization. It should be used in people who are already receiving nitrates, beta-blockers, and CCBs but are still significantly limited by angina. Although effective in women, ranolazine seems to have less of an effect on angina frequency and exercise tolerance in women compared to men. In addition, there is no evidence that treatment with ranolazine decreases the risk of heart attack or death in men or women.

It has one side effect that is fairly worrying to physicians in that it increases something called the *QT interval*. The QT interval is the amount of time from the beginning of the Q wave until the end of the T wave in an EKG, which itself is a diagrammatic representation of the electrical activity of the heart. When the QT interval is prolonged, people who have this condition are at increased risk for serious abnormal heart rhythms. For this reason, ranolazine is contraindicated in people with a prolonged QT, in people taking other medicines that prolong the QT interval, and in people taking other medicines that can interfere with the enzyme that breaks down ranolazine. Some of these medicines are the antifungal ketoconazole,

Table 2–4 Miscellaneous Anti-Anginal

Drug (Trade) Name	Dosage Range (mg/d)
Ranolazine (Ranexa®)	1,000–2,000

verapamil, and diltiazem. It also is contraindicated in people with severe liver disease.

Ranolazine may increase the blood levels of simvastatin and digoxin, so dosages of those medicines may need to be reduced in people on ranolazine.

The most common side effects reported by people who take ranolazine are constipation, headache, dizziness, and nausea. It is usually given twice a day. Table 2–4 shows the daily dosage range and trade name for ranolazine.

CHAPTER 3

Treating Heart Attacks

MYOCARDIAL INFARCTION

Dr. James Herrick in 1912 was the first physician to propose that a clot in a coronary artery led to the clinical picture of *myocardial infarction (MI)*. This is the term doctors give to what lay people call a "heart attack" and it has a very specific medical definition: a myocardial infarction is the death of heart muscle due to interruption of its blood supply. Most MIs are caused by the rupture of an atherosclerotic plaque in a coronary artery. Plaques that have a lot of liquid fat and inflammatory cells are more prone to rupture than plaques that have more scar tissue and less inflammation. When a plaque ruptures and the complex material in the plaque then is exposed to the blood flowing in the artery, the body tries to isolate this material by forming a clot. The plaque material is called *thrombogenic*; that is, it tends to generate or induce the formation of a clot. Physicians, with their love of big words, call such a clot a *thrombosis*. Actually the term thrombosis is used to describe a clot that is *pathologic* (causing disease) whereas a clot that forms when it should, for example, to stop one from bleeding to death from a cut, is termed a *thrombus*. (A clot that breaks off and travels from where it is formed is called an *embolus*.) So the term *coronary thrombosis* sometimes is used to describe the usual cause for a heart attack.

Irreversible injury occurs to heart muscle if blood flow is totally interrupted for more than 20 minutes. The type of MI in which blood flow to the downstream heart muscle is completely cut off, causing injury to the full thickness of muscle making up the wall of the heart, is called an *ST-segment elevation MI (STEMI)* and it is the type with the potential for most heart damage. The name derives from the fact that the EKG of such a person will show elevation of the ST segment of the EKG. Sometimes, however, the clot that is causing the problem does not completely block the artery, and the body's own clot-dissolving molecules often attack the clot and cause it to shrink. In that situation, there just may be frequent episodes of chest pain, which respond to nitroglycerin temporarily, but then recur. The EKG does not show ST-segment elevation (instead it usually shows ST-segment depression, or the T waves may go from being upright to becoming inverted) and this clinical picture is referred to as an *acute coronary syndrome (ACS)*.

In the setting of an STEMI, there is about a 4- to 6-hour window of opportunity during which, if normal blood flow is restored, there will be major salvage of heart muscle and little resulting damage. The main thing that determines the outcome after a MI is how much damage occurs to the heart muscle. If a substantial amount of the heart muscle dies, the result is often chronic congestive heart failure.

About 800,000 people in the United States suffer a MI each year, of whom about one-quarter die. Half of those who die do so before ever reaching the hospital, within an hour or so of first experiencing symptoms. The classic symptoms of MI include crushing substernal (under the breast bone) chest pain, accompanied by breathlessness, sweating, and a feeling of impending doom. This is certainly true of most men who are experiencing a heart attack. However, women may have symptoms that are atypical. They are more apt to have *silent infarctions* than men; that is, MIs with no chest pain at all. They are more apt to have pain in other locations, such as the back, upper abdomen, jaw, and shoulders, and they are more apt to experience severe fatigue and weakness. However, anyone who fears they may be suffering a heart attack should call 911 immediately and be taken to the nearest emergency room, because most heart attacks can be nipped in the bud if they are caught early and treated appropriately. It's important not to be in denial if you are having symptoms that might be from a heart attack. Ignoring them might just be a fatal error and if they turn out to be something else, you, your family, and your doctor will all be relieved.

The acute treatment of MIs involves rapid restoration of blood flow in the affected coronary artery, preferably with a procedure called *percutaneous coronary intervention (PCI)*, with (usually) the insertion of a wire mesh called a *stent* to keep the artery open and provide a scaffold for new tissue to grow and heal the artery. In remote areas that don't have access to the specialized cardiac catheterization laboratories where PCI and stenting are performed, a class of medicines called *thrombolytics* or "clot busters" can be administered intravenously in an attempt to dissolve the offending thrombosis. If thrombolytics are used, they often are followed by the administration of other intravenous blood thinners such as heparin or a class of medicines called *GP IIb IIIa inhibitors*. These intravenous medications will not be discussed further.

However, there also are oral medications that are used in the treatment of MIs. Many of these drugs have already been discussed or will be discussed in the chapters on preventing atherosclerotic cardiovascular disease and treating angina, high blood pressure, or congestive heart failure. Medicines used in the treatment of myocardial infarctions fall into the following categories:

1. Vasodilators including nitrates and ACE inhibitors
2. Antithrombotics, including aspirin and clopidogrel (and warfarin in selected situations)
3. Beta-blockers
4. Cholesterol-lowering medicines, predominantly statins
5. Aldosterone blockers

Someone diagnosed with an acute MI is immediately given 160 to 325 mg of aspirin to chew and swallow unless there is a very strong contraindication such as a history of aspirin allergy or active bleeding into the stomach or bowel. Additional nitroglycerin is usually given either in pill form or intravenously unless the blood pressure is too low (less than 90 mm of mercury systolic) or the heart rate is very rapid or very slow. Long-acting nitrates generally are not used in the setting of acute MI. Oxygen usually is given by nasal tubes, particularly if there is shortness of breath or evidence of lung congestion.

Pain and anxiety almost always are present in people having MIs so morphine is given, usually intravenously.

Many studies have demonstrated that beta-blockers improve the outcome for people with MIs. They usually are started within the first 12 hours, unless the blood pressure or pulse is too low, or there is evidence of severe congestive heart failure.

The medicines that have been proven to be beneficial in this setting include atenolol and metoprolol, which are the only two approved by the FDA for this use in the United States. Treatment with these drugs in the setting of acute MI has been shown to decrease the risk of ventricular fibrillation and atrial fibrillation. They also lower the incidence of progression from impending infarction to completed infarction and reduce the risk of recurrent attacks of angina and infarction in the ensuing six weeks.

The protective effect of beta-blockers in the setting of acute MI is thought to be a class effect, limited however to those that do not also stimulate sympathetic activity, such as pindolol (Visken®), acebutolot (Sectral®), and penbutolol (Levatol®). These beta-blockers have intrinsic sympathomimetic activity (see Chapter 1) and are not prescribed for people with an acute MI.

ACE inhibitors are started within the first 24 hours after an STEMI unless there is a strong contraindication. In people who are allergic or intolerant of ACE inhibitors, an angiotensin receptor blocker may be used. A number of studies have shown that ACE inhibitors reduce the risk of cardiac enlargement and the progression to congestive heart failure in people left with significant heart damage after a MI. They also have been shown to lower the risk of having recurrent fatal or nonfatal cardiac events. The ACE inhibitors used in these clinical trials included enalapril, lisinopril, ramipril, trandolapril, and captopril.

Angiotensin receptor blockers have not been studied in humans in the setting of acute MI, but many physicians use them if their patient cannot tolerate an ACE inhibitor. Valsartan (Diovan®) and candesartan (Atacand®) are the two ARBs generally used in people who have suffered a heart attack.

Aldosterone blockers are given to people who've suffered a heart attack if they are already receiving an ACE inhibitor, and have significant heart damage (an ejection fraction of 40 percent or less), or heart failure. The two medicines approved for this use are spironolactone (Aldactone®) and eplerenone (Inspra®). People with significant kidney disease or high blood potassium should not be given these medicines.

In people who are allergic to aspirin, clopidogrel (Plavix®) or ticlopidine (Ticlid®) should be given instead. After a heart attack, in the absence of allergy or contraindication, aspirin is continued indefinitely, in a dose of 75 to 162 mg/day.

If there is concern that a clot has formed inside the heart—as can happen with very large heart attacks, the blood thinner warfarin (Coumadin®) is given to stabilize the clot and make it less likely to break off and travel to another part of the body, such as the brain.

Intensive therapy with statin medicines has been shown to lower the risk of future heart attacks in randomized controlled trials so standard therapy for MI includes treating people with enough statin medicine to lower LDL-C to less than 70 mg/dl.

It goes without saying that any smoker who has a heart attack *must* quit. The wise and caring physician will have a heart-to-heart talk with such a person and use every available means to help the patient overcome their addiction.

It also goes without saying that after a heart attack, it is crucial to eat a heart-healthy diet, lose weight if you are overweight, and, if your doctor recommends, participate in a supervised cardiac rehabilitation program. The ability to interact with other people in the same situation, learn more about your heart and how to take care of it, and exercise with professional supervision helps to lessen the anxiety and depression that often accompanies an MI.

The therapies discussed in this chapter all have contributed to a marked reduction in the risk of dying from a heart attack for those who make it to a hospital. The chance of dying in hospital before the introduction of coronary care units in the 1960s was about 30 percent. Nowadays, it is about 6 or 7 percent. These advances have been due to the hard work of hundreds of physicians and scientists, and the courage and trust of the many thousands of ordinary people who volunteered their time and effort to participate in clinical trials to determine effective therapies.

CHAPTER 4

Treating Congestive Heart Failure

CONGESTIVE HEART FAILURE

The term *congestive heart failure* (*CHF*) refers to a condition in which the heart cannot pump enough blood around the body to meet the body's needs. The hallmark symptom that people experience with CHF is shortness of breath, what doctors call *dyspnea*. At first, this dyspnea is experienced only during exercise or emotional stress, but in advanced CHF, dyspnea may be present at rest. It also may awaken a person who is suffering from CHF all night, a symptom known as *paroxysmal nocturnal dyspnea* or *PND*. People experiencing PND have to sit on the edge of the bed or stand up in order to breathe more easily. The shortness of breath that occurs in CHF usually is worse when people lie down, a symptom doctors call *orthopnea*. People with this symptom have to sleep propped up on several pillows or in a recliner. An abnormal accumulation of fluid in the lungs causes shortness of breath in CHF. When the fluid accumulation is severe, doctors call it *pulmonary edema*; this condition can be fatal if it is not reversed.

The syndrome of CHF is divided into two main types, depending on whether it is caused by weakness of the heart muscle (*systolic dysfunction*) or increased stiffness of the heart muscle (*diastolic dysfunction*). To find out whether heart failure is due to systolic or diastolic dysfunction, doctors often order a test to determine something called the *ejection fraction*. This is the fraction of blood in the heart during diastole (when the heart is relaxing) that gets ejected during systole (when the heart is contracting). The normal ejection fraction is 55 percent or more. The ejection fraction can be determined from an ultrasound examination of the heart (an *echocardiogram*), by a nuclear scan, by *cardiac magnetic resonance imaging (MRI)*, or by an angiogram.

There are many potential causes for the heart muscle to be weakened. In this country, the most common cause is a heart attack (MI) in which heart muscle dies because its blood supply has been interrupted. Although the heart heals after an MI, the resulting scar tissue cannot contract as normal heart muscle does. If too much heart muscle is replaced with scar tissue, the heart becomes progressively weaker, and the scarred area can balloon out with each heart beat, forming an *aneurysm*.

Long-standing untreated or poorly controlled high blood pressure eventually leads to stretching and weakening of heart muscle and congestive heart failure. If any of the valves in the heart become severely leaky or severely narrowed, CHF can result. A form of systolic heart failure that only occurs in women is called *peripartum cardiomyopathy*. This fortunately rare condition occurs in the last trimester of pregnancy or in the first few months after giving birth. Viral infections of the heart, a medication used to treat cancer called *doxorubicin*, iron-overload disease, an underactive thyroid gland, parasitic infections of the heart, excessive alcohol intake, and some familial diseases can all lead to systolic dysfunction and CHF. Severe obesity can cause CHF of both the systolic and diastolic varieties. Luckily, substantial weight loss leads to improvement in this form or CHF. Some cases of cardiomyopathy are of unknown origin, what doctors call *idiopathic* to cloak our ignorance in a fancy term.

Diastolic dysfunction can have multiple causes. In diastolic dysfunction, the heart's ability to fill with blood or to relax between beats is impaired. The heart sits in a sac of thin tissue called the *pericardium* and if the pericardium is thickened, it puts pressure on the heart, impeding its filling. The heart muscle becomes abnormally stiff temporarily, in the setting of ischemia, or chronically, in conditions like *amyloidosis*, a disease of unknown cause in which an abnormal protein is deposited in the heart.

The hallmark of diastolic dysfunction is dilatation of the receiving chambers of the heart, the atria. If both ventricles are abnormally stiff, both atria will become dilated. If only the left ventricle is abnormally stiff, the left atrium will become dilated. Dilatation of the atria increases the likelihood of abnormal heart rhythms. As in systolic dysfunction, the most common symptom of diastolic dysfunction is shortness of breath.

A frequent accompaniment of dyspnea in people with either form of CHF is an abnormal accumulation of fluid in the legs, called *peripheral edema*. There are many conditions other than CHF that can cause edema or swelling in the legs. The most common is varicose veins. Peripheral edema also can occur in severe kidney or liver disease, if the leg veins are obstructed; for example, by a clot, or if there is anything causing obstruction to venous or lymphatic flow.

In the "old" days, edema used to be called *dropsy* and for centuries, dropsy was treated with an extract of the foxglove plant. The Latin botanical name for the foxglove is *digitalis purpurea*, from which the name of the earliest medicine, used to treat CHF, digitalis, is derived.

The first doctor to write about the use of digitalis in treating dropsy was William Withering. Withering was a graduate of the medical school at the University of Edinburgh. Originally from Shropshire in England, he knew that a popular folk remedy for dropsy or swelling was an extract of foxglove leaves, taken as a tea. He realized that dropsy could be due to heart disease. Withering's "An Account of the Foxglove," which was published in 1785, is one of the classics of clinical medicine. In it, he summarized over 10 years of careful study of the drug digitalis, the cardiac glycoside obtained from the leaves of the foxglove. He advised careful use of digitalis as an effective treatment for dropsy.

Care is needed because in higher doses, digitalis is a poison. When someone has accumulated toxic levels of digitalis in the blood, the first symptom often is loss of appetite, followed by nausea, vomiting, and abdominal pain. Sometimes people with digitalis toxicity see yellow halos around objects, what doctors call *xanthopsia*, but this symptom is rare. People with toxic levels of digitalis in their bodies are also prone to several different kinds of abnormal heart rhythms, some of which can be fatal.

The most commonly prescribed form of digitalis is called *digoxin*. There are drugs that increase the level of digoxin when they are used at the same time. These include quinidine, verapamil, amiodarone, ranolazine, cyclosporine, and spironolactone. The dose of digoxin may need to be reduced in people being treated with these medicines. In addition, because it is excreted by the kidney, the dose of digoxin must be lowered in people with poor kidney function and in the elderly. Low levels of potassium and magnesium, which can occur in people taking diuretics or experiencing diarrhea, also increase the risk of digitalis toxicity.

Digitalis works by increasing the strength of the heart's contraction. Despite being in use for centuries, and many clinical observations as to its ability to improve the shortness of breath and edema associated with CHF, digitalis wasn't studied in randomized controlled trials until the 20th century. These studies confirmed the usefulness of digitalis (most often in the form of digoxin, a relatively short-acting digitalis preparation). Two of these trials confirmed that withdrawing digoxin in people in heart failure led to a worsening of their symptoms and a lessening of their ability to exercise.

In 1997, the results of the Digitalis Investigation Group (DIG) trial were published in the *New England Journal of Medicine*. This study had two substudies: one in people with systolic dysfunction, defined as ejection fractions of 45 percent or less and the other in people with preserved heart muscle function and ejection fractions of more than 45 percent. The DIG trial showed that adding digoxin to standard therapy for CHF (ACE inhibitors and diuretics) in people with depressed ejection fractions did not affect the chance of dying from CHF but did lower the rate of hospitalizations for CHF.

In addition to its use in CHF, digoxin often is prescribed to lower the heart rate in a common abnormal heart rhythm called *atrial fibrillation*. Digoxin usually is given once a day, although in people with kidney disease it is sometimes given every other day, or three times a week. Table 4–1 lists the most commonly prescribed digitalis preparation.

Table 4–1 Digitalis

Drug (Trade Name)	Dosage Range (mg/d)
Digoxin (Lanoxin®)	0.0625–0.25

Diuretics

Historically, diuretics were the next class of medicines to be used to treat CHF after digitalis. The earliest diuretic was Mercuhydrin, which was introduced in the 1930s and was still being used to treat CHF in the late 1960s. It was not particularly effective, had to be injected, and was soon superseded by the more powerful loop diuretics. The retention of excess sodium and water in the body that occurs in CHF is a result of a complex series of adjustments the body makes when the heart is not pumping sufficient blood for its needs. As the left ventricle fails, there is activation of both the sympathetic nervous system (see Chapter 1) and the RAAS (Renin-angiotensin-aldosterone system). The sympathetic nervous system hormones increase the strength of contraction of the failing heart muscle and the RAAS hormones increase the blood volume in an attempt to maintain blood flow to the tissues. Although these responses are effective in the short term, in the long term, they lead to such adverse effects as edema, lung congestion, abnormal thickening of heart muscle, heart muscle cell loss, and a downward spiral leading to death.

The loop diuretics are helpful in ridding the body of excess sodium and water but do nothing to combat the effects of the activation of the RAAS. Studies now have shown that adding diuretics that inhibit the action of aldosterone actually prolong life in people with CHF due to systolic dysfunction. A study published in the *New England Journal of Medicine* in 1999 showed that when the aldosterone antagonist spironolactone was added to usual therapy consisting of ACE inhibitors, loop diuretics, and digoxin, the death rate for people with systolic heart failure was significantly lowered by 30 percent and the rate of hospitalization for CHF also was lowered, by 35 percent.

In another study published in the same journal in 2003, the newest aldosterone antagonist, eplerenone was investigated in people with poor heart function that resulted from an MI. In this study, the risk of death was decreased by 15 percent in people treated with standard therapy plus eplerenone compared to standard therapy plus placebo, and hospitalizations for CHF also were reduced.

People who have poor kidney function may develop dangerously high potassium levels on these medicines so they should not be given to people with significant kidney disease. Eplerenone should not be taken by people on certain other drugs including the antibiotics troleandomycin and clarithromycin, some antifungal medicines, and some HIV medicines. Thiazide diuretics are rarely used alone in treating CHF but are often added for people who have become relatively refractory to the effects of loop diuretics. (See Table 1–3 in Chapter 1.) Table 4–2 lists the aldosterone antagonists that are used in the treatment of CHF.

BETA-BLOCKERS

When beta-blockers were first introduced in the 1960s, it was thought that they would make people with CHF worse. However, studies undertaken in the 1990s proved that when used in people with heart failure, beta-blockers actually made people feel better and live longer. More than 20 trials involving about 6000 peo-

Table 4–2 Aldosterone Antagonists

Drug (Trade Name)	Dosage Range(mg/d)
Spironolactone (Aldactone®)	12.5–100
Eplerenone (Inspra®)	25–50

ple showed a lowering of the risk of death, fewer hospitalizations, less progression of heart failure, and improved heart function when beta-blockers were added to therapy with ACE inhibitors and diuretics. Currently, unless there is a very strong contraindication, or someone has been unable to tolerate treatment with them, all people with CHF are prescribed a beta-blocker.

There are three beta-blockers that have been shown to be effective in the therapy of CHF. They are bisoprolol, metoprolol, and carvedilol. Of these three medicines, only carvedilol blocks both beta and alpha receptors.

In a trial conducted in Europe between 1996 and 1999, people with CHF were randomized to receive either carvedilol or long-acting metoprolol tartrate. In this study of over 3000 patients followed for an average of 58 months, those treated with carvedilol had a 34 percent death rate compared to a 40 percent death rate for those treated with long-acting metoprolol. The likelihood of either dying or needing hospitalization was not different between the two groups. However, the metoprolol tartrate used in that study (marketed in the United States as Lopressor) is not identical with the metoprolol succinate which is approved in this country for treating CHF.

People with severely decreased heart muscle function should not receive beta-blockers until they are on the other standard medicines for CHF (ACE inhibitors or ARBs) and have received diuretics to remove excess fluid. They then are started on low doses of beta-blockers, with the dose increased every two weeks as tolerated. Sometimes it is necessary to take higher doses of diuretics while the dose of beta-blockers is being increased. In general, beta-blockers are not used to treat people with brittle, insulin-dependent diabetes (the beta-blockers can mask the symptoms of low blood sugar). In addition, people with abnormally slow heart rates, severe asthma, and serious arterial disease in the arteries to the legs usually cannot be treated with beta-blockers.

Long-acting metoprolol is generally given once a day. The dose should be titrated up from 25 mg daily to 200 mg daily, if tolerated. Carvedilol initially needed to be taken twice a day but more recently a new preparation, called Coreg CR, has become available and can be taken once a day. The dose of carvedilol, depending on which preparation is used, should be titrated up from 3.25 mg twice a day to 25 mg twice a day for the twice-daily preparation, or from 10 mg a day to 80 mg a day for the once-daily preparation. Carvedilol needs to be taken with meals. Bisoprolol is taken once a day, in an initial dose of 1.25 mg a day, increasing to 10 mg a day if tolerated.

Table 4–3 lists the beta-blocker preparations that are approved to treat CHF in the United States.

Table 4–3 Beta Blockers for CHF

Drug (Trade) Name	Dosage Range (mg/d)
Bisoprolol (Zebeta®)	1.25–10
Carvedilol (Coreg®)	6.25–50
Carvedilol (Coreg CR®)	10–80
Metoprolol succinate (Toprol XL®)	25–200

ACE INHIBITORS

Angiotensin-converting enzyme (ACE) was discovered in 1956 but the first angiotensin-converting enzyme inhibitor was not synthesized until 1975. This medicine, captopril, was approved by the FDA to treat high blood pressure in 1981. Although they were first introduced to treat high blood pressure, the beneficial effects of this class of medicines for CHF became apparent through a series of clinical trials that were undertaken in the last few decades.

In addition to dilating arteries, which lessens the work the failing heart muscle has to perform, ACE inhibitors also influence the negative effects that occur when the RAAS is activated in CHF. Multiple clinical trials have demonstrated that adding ACE inhibition to the standard therapy of digoxin and diuretics lowers the death and hospitalization rates in CHF. Some patients cannot tolerate ACE inhibitors, either because of allergic reactions, cough, or kidney failure, but in general, except in those circumstances, people who have CHF should be treated with one of these medicines. As noted previously, they should not be used in women who are pregnant.

Table 4–4 lists the ACE inhibitors that are approved for the treatment of CHF in the United States. Captopril is taken in divided doses, three times a day an hour before meals. Quinapril and ramipril can be taken twice daily. Enalapril, lisinopril, and trandolapril can be taken once daily.

Table 4–4 Angiotensin Converting Enzyme Inhibitors for CHF

Drug (Trade) Name	Dosage Range (mg/d)
Captopril (Capoten®)	18.75–300
Enalapril (Vasotec®)	2.5–40
Fosinopril (Monopril®)	5–40
Lisinopril (Prinivil, Zestril®)	5–40
Perindopril (Aceon®)	2–16
Quinapril (Accupril®)	10–40
Ramipril (Altace®)	2.5–10
Trandolapril (Mavik®)	1–4

ANGIOTENSIN RECEPTOR BLOCKERS

Some people cannot take ACE inhibitors, either because of a bothersome cough or the development of an allergic reaction. At other times, people may develop a tolerance to ACE inhibitors, which means they lose their effectiveness. In those instances, ARBs may be used in place of ACE inhibitors to treat people with CHF.

Like ACE inhibitors, the beneficial effect of some of the ARBs has been confirmed by clinical trials. The two ARBs that are approved for use in treating CHF in this country are candesartan and valsartan. Candesartan® is given once a day, and valsartan is given twice a day to people with CHF. These medicines usually are started at a low dose, with doubling of the dose every two weeks, if tolerated, until the maximum dose is achieved. Just as with ACE inhibitors, ARBs may cause kidney failure, high levels of potassium, and allergic reactions. They are less likely than ACE inhibitors to cause coughing and must not be given to pregnant women because of the risk of fetal harm or death. Table 4–5 lists the ARBs approved for use in CHF.

MISCELLANEOUS THERAPIES FOR CHF

Even before ACE inhibitors were shown to be effective in the treatment of CHF, an earlier clinical trial showed that treating men with damaged heart muscle with a combination of the blood vessel dilator hydralazine (see Chapter 1 in the section on treating hypertension), and the long-acting nitrate isosorbide (see Chapter 2 in the section on long-acting oral nitrates) was effective in lowering the risk of death. This study was done in Veteran's Administration hospitals and was called the Vasodilator Heart Failure Trial (V-HeFT). The results were reported in 1986. When the authors analyzed the results by ethnicity, they found that African-American men derived an even greater benefit than Caucasian men from this combination therapy.

Subsequent studies showed that African Americans had less blood pressure lowering when they were treated with ACE inhibitors and did not appear to derive as much benefit as Caucasians when they were treated with ACE inhibitors for CHF. The African-American Heart Failure Trial (A-HeFT) was designed to learn if treatment with a fixed-dose combination of hydralazine and isosorbide added to standard therapy with an ACE inhibitor/ARB, diuretics, and the like, improved the

Table 4–5 Angiotensin Receptor Blockers for CHF

Drug (Trade) Name	Dosage Range (mg/d)
Candesartan (Atacand®)	4–32
Losartan (Cozaar®)	25–100
Valsartan (Diovan®)	40–320

Table 4–6 Combination Therapy for CHF

Drug (Trade) Name	Dosage Range (mg)
Hydralazine/isosorbide (Bidil)	37.5/20 three times daily

Table 4–7

Generic (Trade) Name	Dosage Range (mg/d)
Bromocriptine (Parlodel)	2.5–5

outcome in 1050 African-American men and women with severe heart failure. The study was begun in 2001 and stopped prematurely for benefit in 2004. (When a clinical trial shows a significant benefit of the medicine being studied before the planned end date of the trial, the study is stopped and all participants are told of the results and given the opportunity to take the active medicine.) Survival was increased by 43 percent in the people who received active drugs compared to placebo in A-HeFT. The participants on active drug also required fewer hospitalizations and had a better quality of life.

As a result of this trial, a fixed dose combination pill containing 37.5 mg of hydralazine and 20 mg of isosorbide dinitrate was introduced in 2005 as the first FDA heart failure pill designed specifically for African-American patients. The pill is added to standard therapy and needs to be taken three times a day. The most common side effects are headache and dizziness, and because the pills contain a nitrate, any of the drugs for erectile dysfunction cannot be taken within 24 hours. Table 4–6 lists this medication and its daily dosage range.

The treatment of CHF has been revolutionized in the past few decades. In addition to whole new classes of medicine, people with advanced heart failure now have access to cardiac transplantation, and in some instances, a special pacemaker, called a *biventricular pacemaker*, which can improve heart function and prolong life. William Withering would be astounded and no doubt pleased at the progress his medical descendants have made in treating this debilitating condition.

CHAPTER 5

Treating Abnormal Heart Rhythms

NORMAL HEART RHYTHMS

People often refer to their heart as "my ticker." This is not a bad description because, in addition to being a muscular pump, the heart has its own electrical system that prompts it to beat in a steady rhythm. When the normal organized electrical activity in the heart is interfered with, an abnormal heart rhythm, what doctors call an *arrhythmia* can result. In some instances, this causes people to feel their heart skipping or beating unusually fast or slow. The term used to describe this sensation is *palpitations*. In the worst-case scenario, disorganized electrical activity in the heart may cause a rapidly fatal arrhythmia called *ventricular fibrillation*.

Normally, the electrical impulse that prompts the heart muscle to contract begins in a little area high in the right atrium called the *sinus node* or *sinoatrial node (SAN)*. The normal heart rhythm is called *normal sinus rhythm*. The SAN sends out an electrical impulse at a rate between 60 and 100 times per minute, depending on a person's age and level of activity (or anxiety). The impulse travels through both the right and left atria, causing the muscles of the atria to squeeze. When this happens, the tricuspid and mitral valves open, allowing blood to flow from the atria to the ventricles. The impulse gets held up for part of a second in another structure called the *atrio-ventricular node (AVN)*, which sits low in the wall or septum that divides the right and left atria. From there, the electrical impulse travels through specialized fibers called the *His-Purkinje system* to both the ventricles, causing them to contract and eject blood out through the pulmonic and aortic valves to the pulmonary artery and aorta. Figure 5–1 depicts the electrical conducting system of the heart.

The electrical activity of the heart can be measured and displayed on paper. This is the well-known test called an *electrocardiogram* or *EKG*. Figure 5–2 displays the electrical activity of the heart during one heartbeat. The P wave is caused by the electrical impulse traveling through the atria, the QRS complex is caused by the electrical stimulation of the ventricles, and the T wave is caused by the ventricles recovering, or "repolarizing" so that they can be stimulated again. The time it takes for the electrical impulse to travel through the atria and AV node causes the PR interval, and the time it takes for the ventricles to become stimulated and then recover causes the QT interval.

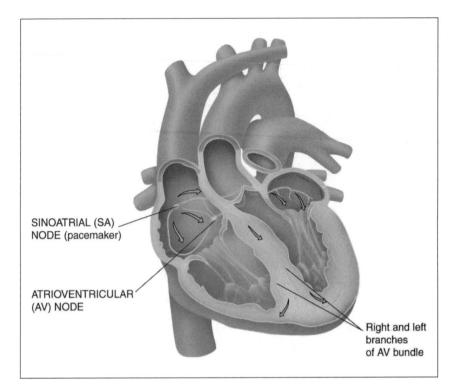

SINOATRIAL (SA)
NODE (pacemaker)

ATRIOVENTRICULAR
(AV) NODE

Right and left
branches
of AV bundle

Figure 5–1 Electrical conducting system of the heart: The conduction system of the heart. These specializes groups of cardiac muscle cells initiate an electrical impulse through the heart, beginning in the sinoartial (SA) node and spreading to the atrioventricular (AV) node. The AV node then initiates a signal that is conducted through the ventricles.
Courtesy of Jones & Bartlett

Abnormal heart rhythms can be classified by whether they are too fast or too slow (*tachycardia* or *bradycardia*) or they can be classified by their site of origin (atrial or ventricular). There are no medicines that can be taken chronically by mouth to correct a heart rate that is too slow. The treatment for bradycardia which is causing symptoms (and not arising from medication or some correctable cause like an underactive thyroid) is a pacemaker, a device that takes over for the sinus node. When we talk about treating abnormal heart rhythms therefore, we are talking about treating tachycardias, rhythms that are too fast. The tachycardias can be classified by whether they arise in the atria or AVN (supraventricular) or in the ventricles (ventricular).

Before getting into the treatment of the various abnormal heart rhythms, a discussion of palpitations may clear up some misconceptions about this symptom.

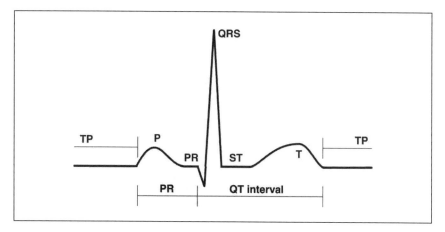

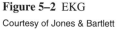

Figure 5–2 EKG
Courtesy of Jones & Bartlett

PALPITATIONS

Palpitations are a very common complaint among patients referred to cardiologists. In fact, chest pain or palpitations are the two most common symptoms described by the majority of patients who are referred to me. Defined as a "rapid, violent or throbbing pulsation, as an abnormally rapid throbbing or fluttering of the heart" palpitations usually are caused by an irregularity in the heart's rhythm. Some people never experience the sensation of a fluttering in the chest, despite having so-called "extra beats" whereas others are deeply attuned to every perturbation in their heart's rhythm. Figure 5–3 shows an EKG tracing from someone having what

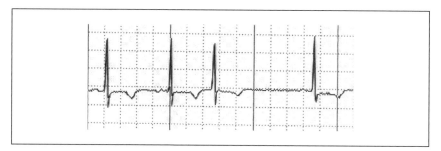

Figure 5–3 EKG tracing from someone having what doctors refer to as a *premature atrial contraction (PAC)*

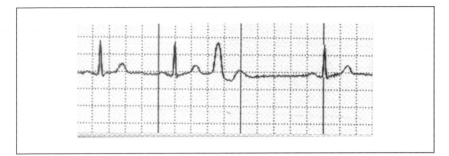

Figure 5–4 EKG tracing from someone having what doctors refer to as a *premature ventricular contraction (PVC)*.

---

doctors refer to as a *premature atrial contraction (PAC)*. Figure 5–4 shows what is referred to as a *premature ventricular contraction (PVC)*.

You can see that there is a pause after each of these premature beats. During this pause, the heart fills with more blood than usual, and the beat after the pause is more forceful than normal. It is actually this beat that people usually sense when they have a palpitation. If your palpitations are not associated with other symptoms such as severe dizziness, fainting, shortness of breath, or chest pain, they are almost certainly benign.

In the absence of diagnosed heart disease, premature contractions are not cause for concern. Even young healthy people with perfectly normal hearts have premature contractions—however, they are more apt to occur in the setting of heart disease and in certain other situations. An underactive or overactive thyroid can cause extra beats (usually ventricular in the former and atrial in the latter case); caffeine, decongestants, cocaine use, alcohol abuse, and low blood potassium or magnesium all increase the likelihood of extra beats. As part of the investigation of palpitations, your doctor will try to exclude these factors.

To determine if extra beats are causing palpitations, physicians often order a test called a *24-hour Holter monitor*. EKG electrodes are placed on your chest and hooked up to a small portable recording device that can be worn around the waist. You will be instructed to keep a diary of any symptoms and your activity, over the 24 hours of the recording. The EKG tracing then will be analyzed to determine if your symptom of palpitations coincides with an irregularity of the heart rhythm. If you are found to have isolated premature contractions as a cause of your palpitations, your doctor probably will just reassure you and urge you to ignore them. If they are very frequent or bothersome to you, your doctor may prescribe beta-blockers for PVCs or diltiazem or verapamil for PACs.

The important thing to remember about palpitations is that in people without heart disease, they are almost always benign and don't carry an ominous prognosis.

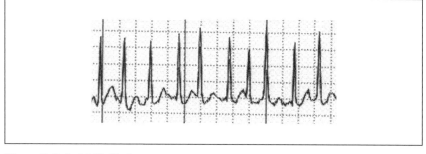

Figure 5–5 Atrial fibrillation

SUPRAVENTRICULAR ARRHYTHMIAS

The most common supraventricular tachycardia is *atrial fibrillation (AF)*, accounting for about 35 percent of arrhythmias in people who are hospitalized. In this condition, the atria beat in a very rapid disorganized fashion; in fact, they appear to be quivering, not beating, at rates exceeding 300 per minute. The AVN gets bombarded with these electrical impulses, most of which don't get through, but those that do cause the ventricles to beat in an irregularly irregular fashion, and usually at rates above 100 per minute. This causes the electrocardiogram to have a characteristic appearance. Figure 5–5 illustrates an example of atrial fibrillation.

The likelihood of developing AF increases with age. In people who are 50 to 59 years of age, about 1 in 200 will have this condition, but in people in their 80s, about 9 per 100 have AF. Certain conditions other than age predispose to developing AF; these include an overactive thyroid, high blood pressure, coronary artery disease, congestive heart failure, and valvular heart disease. If AF has been present for years, it is unlikely that either an electrical shock to the heart, called *cardioversion*, or medication will be able to terminate it. The shorter the time that AF has been present, and the less diseased the heart is, the better the chance that AF can be converted to NSR.

Some people who have AF have no symptoms at all. Others may be aware of their heart beating rapidly or irregularly. They may feel short of breath, dizzy, lightheaded, and may experience chest discomfort. People with AF may have it because their thyroid is overactive, or because of problems with leaky or narrowed heart valves. Sometimes people who binge drink develop episodes of AF. These precipitating causes should be looked for in anyone who develops AF.

The most feared complication of AF is a stroke. This comes about because without organized contractions; the blood in the atria tends to stagnate and stagnant blood is more apt to clot than blood that is flowing normally. If a clot forms in the left atrium, it can break off and travel to other parts of the body. If a clot travels to the brain, it can cause a stroke. Ideally then, doctors like to keep people in normal sinus rhythm and out of atrial fibrillation. If that cannot be accomplished, then people who have AF, whether it is continuous or intermittent, should be treated with the blood thinner warfarin (Coumadin®) that has been proven to lower the risk of stroke. There are some exceptions to this recommendation; for example, people who have a history of life-threatening bleeding, and in some low-risk younger people (under the age of 65) with only very brief episodes of AF, and no other risk factors for stroke (such as hypertension, valvular disease, or a very enlarged left atrium). In these low-risk people, aspirin can be used to lower the risk of clotting instead of warfarin. In people who have a very strong reason for not being on blood thinners, another treatment option is to do a special test called a *transesophageal echocardiogram*. In this test, a flexible tube is inserted into the esophagus, the tube leading from the mouth to the stomach. An ultrasound transducer is incorporated into this tube and takes ultrasound pictures of the left atrium. This is an accurate way of finding out if there is a clot in the left atrium. If there isn't a clot, then it is safe to try to electrically convert AF to a normal sinus rhythm without thinning the blood.

Sometimes AF is well tolerated but there are certain heart conditions in which the occurrence of AF can lead to fainting or worsening CHF. On rare occasions, people who go into AF, especially if their heart rate is very rapid, may go into shock and in this situation, the physician probably will apply an electrical shock to the chest (after putting the patient to sleep) to stop the AF. However, this procedure, *direct current electrocardioversion*, is most often done electively, after treatment to thin the blood for several weeks.

Some medicines are effective in slowing the heart rate in AF and there are others that can convert AF to normal sinus rhythm and lessen the likelihood that AF will recur. The first group includes the old standbys digoxin, beta-blockers, and the nondihydropyridine CCBs diltiazem and verapamil. These medicines slow the heart rate in atrial fibrillation but are unlikely to convert it to normal sinus rhythm. They often are used temporarily until a cardioversion can be performed, generally after treatment with warfarin for 3 to 4 weeks. If someone has been in atrial fibrillation for less than 48 hours, it is felt safe to cardiovert without thinning the blood for 3 to 4 weeks. However, if AF has been present for more than 48 hours or when it is unknown how long it has been present, then no attempt to convert the rhythm back to a normal sinus rhythm is made until the blood has been thinned. The only exception to this is if the AF is causing the blood pressure to drop to dangerous levels, which generally occurs only rarely in people with serious heart conditions.

The oral medicines that can be used to convert AF to NSR, include amiodarone, dofetilide, flecainide, and propafenonel. These same medicines, plus sotalol and disopyramide may be prescribed to maintain sinus rhythm after AF has been converted, with medication or electrical cardioversion. All of these medicines carry a risk of causing side effects; the most serious of which is something called *proarrhythmia*, the occurrence of another abnormal heart rhythm caused by the medicine used to treat the first abnormal heart rhythm. The most serious proarrhythmia is called *torsades de pointes* and it can be fatal. This complication is more apt to occur in people who have a prolonged QT interval (see previous information on page 57), so if a prolonged QT is present, drug therapy is probably not a good idea.

Flecainide and propafenone may be used in people who have no heart condition other than AF, but should be avoided in people with coronary artery disease, damaged heart muscle, or CHF. For such people, these medicines carry an unacceptably high risk of proarrhythmia. Flecainide usually is taken twice a day without regard to meals, starting with a lower dose and increasing every four days until the standard daily dose is achieved. It can cause constipation, nausea, loss of appetite, headache, dizziness, and rash. Propafenone usually is taken every eight hours and the dose is increased gradually at about four-day intervals until the usual daily dose is reached. Propafenone may cause people to experience an unusual taste in the mouth, constipation, nausea, dizziness, headaches, and weakness. Flecainide and propafenone usually are given with a beta-blocker because sometimes they cause AF to change into atrial flutter, another arrthymia, and if this happens, the heart rate can become even faster. The beta-blocker makes this less likely to happen.

In the past, another medicine, quinidine was often used to treat AF. Quinidine was effective in the short term but its long-term use was associated with significant risks of proarrhythmia and even an increased risk of death. This was found on analyzing the results of seven studies in which quinidine was used in AF. Quinidine also can cause platelets to drop to levels that can cause serious bleeding. (*Platelets* are little formed elements of the blood taht are crucial in clotting.) Quinidine frequently causes nausea and diarrhea. For these reasons, quinidine is no longer used in the treatment of AF.

Disopyramide is similar to quinidine in its actions and is safer when given chronically quinidine. It comes in a shorter-acting form that needs to be taken four times a day and a long-acting form that can be taken twice a day. However, disopyramide has certain side effects that sometimes make it difficult to tolerate. It may cause difficulty with urination in men with enlarged prostates and can cause worsening of glaucoma and dry mouth. Disopyramide also decreases the force of the heart muscle contraction and can therefore increase CHF in people with a damaged left ventricle. This latter action of disopyramide makes it potentially useful sometimes in a condition called *hypertrophic obstructive cardiomyopathy (HOCM)* in which lessening the force of contraction is a desired effect, in order to decrease the obstruction to ventricular emptying that occurs in HOCM.

Sotalol has beta-blocking activity but in other respects is like amiodarone and dofetilide. Because of a significant risk of proarrhythmia, sotalol generally is started in the hospital where continuous EKG monitoring is available to detect any adverse effects. Monitoring should continue for a minimum of three days. Sotalol usually is given twice a day. It should not be used in people with a prolonged QT, and low blood potassium should be corrected before this medicine is given. In common with other beta-blocking agents, sotalol may worsen asthma and cause fatigue and an abnormal slowing of the heart rate.

Like sotalol, dofetilide should be started in the hospital with continuous EKG monitoring for at least three days to detect proarrhythmia. If low blood potassium is present, it must be corrected before using this drug. The dosage needs to be carefully calculated based on the kidney function of the person being treated. People with very depressed kidney function, or prolongation of the QT interval should not be treated with dofetilide. Dofetilide is usually taken twice daily. Headache, chest pain, and dizziness sometimes are reported by people taking dofetilide.

Amiodarone is the drug used most commonly to maintain people who have had an episode of AF in a normal rhythm. It originally was developed to treat angina, because one of its effects is to dilate blood vessels. It was not long before doctors noted that it also had a beneficial effect on abnormal heart rhythms. Amiodarone was used in Europe for more than 20 years before it was approved in the United States in 1985. It has a low likelihood of causing proarrythmia, but it has many other potential side effects. It can cause serious lung damage, thyroid disease, hepatitis (inflammation of the liver), sun sensitivity, bluish discoloration of the skin, inflammation of the optic (eye) nerve, and deposits in the cornea of the eye. People also may experience nausea, constipation, loss of appetite, fatigue, tremors, and malaise. Some of these side effects are dose dependent but others, like lung disease, can occur quite soon after beginning treatment.

People who have been on stable doses of warfarin who are then treated with amiodarone must have their warfarin dose reduced and blood tests checked more frequently because their blood may become too thin if they are maintained on the same dose of warfarin. The dose of warfarin should be cut by one-third to one-half when amiodarone is started to avoid the risk of serious bleeding. Amiodarone must be used with caution in people taking beta-blockers, diltiazem, or verapamil, because the pulse may drop to dangerously low levels. Digoxin levels also increase in people put on amiodarone, so the digoxin dose should be cut in half when amiodarone is used to avoid digitalis toxicity.

Certain other drugs, including some HIV medicines, the antidepressant trazadone, cimetidine (Tagamet®), and large amounts of grapefruit juice can cause increased levels of amiodarone when they are taken together.

It takes weeks for a steady concentration of amiodarone to build up in the blood so people are often put on a higher "loading" dose for a few weeks in order for the effect to occur in a timely fashion. Once in the body, amiodarone is excreted extremely slowly, over a period of months.

Amiodarone and dofetilide are the only AF drugs that have been shown to be safe for people who have congestive heart failure. Table 5–1 lists the drugs used in the treatment of atrial fibrillation with their usual daily dose range.

Sometimes, no matter what drug therapy is used, AF recurs or cannot be converted in the first place. In this situation, controlling the heart rate (with medicines like digoxin, beta-blockers, diltiazem, or verapamil) and chronic blood thinning with coumadin are very effective in allowing people to live productive, active lives. However, physicians would like to have something better than drugs with all their potential side effects to offer their patients with AF. This has prompted research into new therapies to "cure" AF, some of which are already available in large medical centers.

Table 5–1 Drugs used in Atrial Fibrillation

Drug (Trade) Name	Dosage Range (mg/d)
Amiodarone (Cordarone®, Pacerone®)	100–400 (after loading)
Disopyramide (Norpace, Norpace CR®)	400–800
Dofetilide (Tikosyn®)	0.25–1.0
Flecainide (Tambocor®)	100–300
Propafenone (Rythmol®)	450–900
Propafenone (Rythmol SR®)	450–850
Sotalol (Betapace AF®)	160–320

The newest therapy for AF involves a catheter technique called *ablation* which is only available in specialized *electrophysiologic laboratories* where subspecialty cardiologists called *electrophysiologists* use radiofrequency waves to destroy or isolate the tissue in the atria and pulmonary veins that are responsible for the arrhythmia. However, serious complications can occur with this procedure, including stroke and narrowing of the pulmonary veins, leading to heart failure, It is still considered experimental but as with any other new procedure is likely to be refined, and made safer, as physicians become more skilled at performing it.

There is also a surgical treatment, called the *MAZE procedure*, in which multiple incisions are made in the atrial tissue, which interrupts the propagation of the electrical impulses that result in AF. This is done most often in the situation where someone with AF is undergoing open-heart surgery for some other reason, such as a valve replacement or bypass grafting.

It is likely that ablation procedures will play an increasing role in the treatment of AF. They are already used quite successfully to treat other abnormal heart rhythms that arise in the atria, the AV node, and ventricles. These abnormal rhythms that arise in the upper chambers of the heart are called *atrial tachycardia, atrial flutter*, and *AV nodal tachycardia* (these, along with AF, are collectively referred to as *supraventricular tachycardias, SVT)*. Sometimes these abnormal rhythms occur in people with otherwise normal hearts, and sometimes they occur in people with heart disease.

There is a condition known as *Wolf-Parkinson-White (WPW)* syndrome in which there are extra connections between the atria and ventricles, called *bypass tracts*, over which electrical impulses can travel. People with this syndrome may have AF with a very rapid heart rate, or frequent episodes of SVT. Ablation may be used in this situation because people with WPW may actually increase their heart rates to dangerous levels when treated with medicines that are used safely in people without these bypass tracts.

Unlike the other SVTs, people who experience atrial flutter are thought to be at increased risk of developing clots in the left atrium, similar to the situation with

AF. Therefore, most people with atrial flutter that has lasted more than 48 hours have their blood thinned for 3 to 4 weeks with Coumadin® before an attempt is made to convert them to a normal rhythm either with medicine, ablation, or electrical cardioversion.

Ablation may be used to treat these SVTs when people do not respond to medications, have side effects to medications, or simply don't want to have to take medications indefinitely for a condition that may only occur rarely. Beta-blockers, digoxin, diltiazem, and verapamil often are used to treat SVTs. If someone has SVT only once a year or so, they sometimes can just take medicine on an as needed basis.

VENTRICULAR ARRHYTHMIAS

Ventricular tachycardia (VT) can occur in people with otherwise normal hearts but more commonly occurs in the presence of heart disease, particularly atherosclerotic cardiovascular disease. With VT, the heart rate is rapid (120 beats per minute or more) and the heart's contraction is ineffective, so it is more common for people who experience VT to feel dizzy or even faint, than it is for people who have SVT. People who are diagnosed with VT and have symptoms, particularly if they have documented heart disease, can now be treated with either drugs (usually beta-blockers, amiodarone, or sotalol), ablation, or implantable devices (see the following). Sometimes they are treated with a combination of these therapies. Some types of VT respond to the calcium channel blocker verapamil. Determining the best treatment for VT usually requires referral to an electrophysiologist.

There is a special form of VT called *torsades de pointes* where the EKG looks like a picket fence on hilly terrain. This arrhythmia often is caused by medications that prolong the QT interval so treatment involves stopping these.

Another form of VT, called *right ventricular outflow tract (RVOT)* VT can occur in people with normal hearts. This type of VT usually is not dangerous, but if it causes bothersome palpitations, it can be treated with beta-blockers, calcium channel blockers, or ablation.

Ventricular flutter is a very dangerous arrhythmia in which the electrical impulse that drives the heart arises in the ventricle; the heart rate in ventricular flutter is between 180 and 250 beats per minute. This is too rapid to sustain an adequate flow of blood to the brain so this abnormal rhythm usually causes fainting. It often degenerates into an even more dangerous arrhythmia called *ventricular fibrillation*.

Ventricular fibrillation (VF) is a rapid abnormal rhythm with no regular QRS pattern visible on the EKG. The heart in VF simply quivers, it doesn't contract. When VF occurs, there is no organized pumping action, so blood flow from the heart essentially ceases, and if this arrhythmia is not corrected within four or five minutes, death ensues. VF is the usual abnormal rhythm in people who experience *sudden cardiac death (SCD)*. The treatment of VF is electrical *defibrillation* with a direct electric current of 200 to 400 joules applied to the chest wall.

Coronary artery disease and heart attacks are the most common cause of VF, but any condition that causes damage to the heart muscle increases the likelihood of VF. Sometimes a blow to the chest during a vulnerable part of the heart's electric cycle can cause VF even in healthy people. This is the usual cause of death in young athletes who collapse and die after sustaining a blow to the chest; for example, from a baseball.

People with an inherited disorder called *Long QT syndrome*, low levels of potassium and/or magnesium (which can occur in people on diuretics or with severe diarrhea), people on drugs that prolong the QT interval, and some people with WPW syndrome are at increased risk of VF. People with Long QT syndrome who have VT may be treated effectively with beta-blockers, but not all subtypes of Long QT syndrome respond to beta-blockers and most people with this disorder now are treated with an implantable defibrillator.

The chance of success in aborting VF depends on the underlying cause and on the rapidity with which electrical cardioversion is performed. Because early defibrillation is so crucial to surviving this arrhythmia, *automatic external defibrillators (AEDs)* now are commonly found in public places such as airplanes, schools, and sports arenas. The American Heart Association (AHA) sponsors training sessions for laypeople in the performance of *cardiopulmonary resuscitaion (CPR)* and the use of AEDs. To learn the location of a course in your area, go to the AHA Web site at www.americanheart.org/presenter.jhtml?identifier=3011764 and click on *Find a Class Near You* after entering your zip code.

The development of *automatic implantable cardiac defibrillators (AICDs)* has revolutionized the treatment of VT and VF. These devices are inserted into the right side of the heart via a vein in the chest, and the generator pack which powers the device is inserted under the skin. This procedure usually is performed by an electrophysiologist. There are certain criteria that people must meet before they are considered for an AICD but in general, people who survive an episode of VF and have an ejection fraction below 30 percent are likely to benefit from these devices. AICDs can detect VT and VF when they occur and are programmed to deliver an electric shock to the heart to terminate the arrhythmia. Even with an AICD in place, most people with VT or VF are treated with medicines as well. People who have had a shock from an AICD describe it as feeling like "a kick in the chest." That's not a particularly pleasant sensation so medicines are prescribed to lessen the likelihood that a shock will be needed. Amiodarone, beta-blockers, and sotalol are the drugs most commonly prescribed in this situation. Two other medicines, disopyramide and tocainide, also can be used.

When amiodarone is used in this situation, a loading dose of between 800–1600 mg/day is given for one to three weeks, followed by 600–800 mg/day for a month. After that, the dose is reduced to 200–400 mg/day. These doses should be reduced for elderly patients.

Sotalol is usually started in the hospital under continuous EKG monitoring at a dose of 80 mg twice daily and increased every three days to a dose of 120–160 mg twice daily. Lower doses are given if kidney function is not normal.

Table 5–2 Drugs Used in Conjunction with AICD in VT/VF

Drug (Trade) Name	Dosage Range (mg/d)
Amiodarone (Cordarone®, Pacerone®)	200–400 (after loading)
Sotalol (Betapace®)	160–320

Because most patients with AICDs have low-ejection fractions, they will usually already be on therapy with either metoprolol or carvedilol at the time they receive an AICD.

Table 5–2 shows the drugs that are used, usually in conjunction with an AICD, in people who have VT or who have survived an episode of VF.

CHAPTER 6

Treating Primary Pulmonary Hypertension

PRIMARY PULMONARY HYPERTENSION

To understand this relatively rare condition, we should review some basic anatomy. The *pulmonary* arteries carry venous blood to the lungs, where, in the pulmonary capillaries, carbon dioxide and water vapor are given up and oxygen is taken aboard. The *systemic* arteries carry arterial blood all over the body, where, in the capillaries, oxygen and nutrients are given up and carbon dioxide is taken aboard. When the pressure in the systemic arteries increases above the normal range, this is called high blood pressure, or hypertension. When the pressure in the pulmonary arteries increases above the normal range, this is called *pulmonary hypertension*. Compared to systemic arteries, pulmonary arteries have less smooth muscle in their wall, so they are less predisposed to become hypertensive.

Most instances of pulmonary hypertension are caused by cardiac or pulmonary disease, and the treatment involves treating the underlying cause. These disorders are examples of *secondary pulmonary hypertension*. For example, the pulmonary artery pressure may be elevated acutely if a clot travels from elsewhere in the body and lodges in the lungs, a so-called *pulmonary embolism*. Smokers often develop emphysema, in which tiny air spaces called *alveoli* and their capillaries are destroyed. This too causes the pressure in the pulmonary arteries to increase. Many people with narrowed or leaky mitral or aortic valves also develop secondary pulmonary hypertension, because the left ventricle fails as a result of an increased workload imposed by the faulty valve. An unusual ccause of pulmonary hypertenstion was discovered a few decades ago. Outbreaks of pulmonary hypertension at that time were traced to the drug combination Fen Phen, used as an appetite suppressant in people trying to lose weight. Fen Phen was subsequently taken off the market.

Primary pulmonary hypertension (PPH), while uncommon, it is a distinct disorder of unknown cause, which was until recently, a rapidly lethal condition. PPH affects women, generally between the ages of 10 and 40, more often than men. The most common symptoms are shortness of breath, fatigue, dizziness, palpitations, and fainting, all without obvious cause.

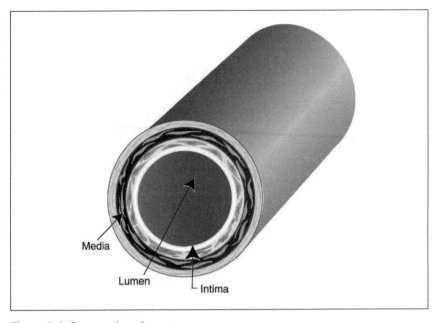

Figure 6–1 Cross section of an artery
Courtesy of Jones & Bartlett

PPH appears to be the result of injury to the wall of the small pulmonary arteries and arterioles (the tiny terminal branches of arteries just before they become capillaries). In response to injury, the innermost layer, called the *intima*, instead of being a layer one cell in depth enlarges and progressively narrows the opening or *lumen* of the artery. The smooth muscle in the next layer, the *media*, also enlarges. Figure 6–1 depicts a normal artery with its lumen intima and media.

The nature of the injury that sets off this response is unknown. However, abnormal clotting is thought to play a role and microscopic study of small pulmonary arteries and arterioles in this condition sometimes reveals clots in these vessels. For this reason, unless there is a very strong contraindication, people with PPH are treated with chronic anticoagulation, usually with warfarin. There is a genetic form of PPH and the gene responsible for these familial cases has been identified.

People who are suspected of having PPH usually undergo a cardiac catheterization, focusing on the right side of the heart. During this test, the response of the pulmonary pressure to various vasodilating drugs is determined. The three most commonly used vasodilators in the catheterization laboratory are inhaled *nitric oxide*, intravenous *adenosine*, and intravenous *prostacyclin*. If the average pulmonary artery pressure falls by 10 mmHg, this is considered a favorable or positive response and such people are more apt to respond to therapy with the CCBs, nifedipine, amlodipine, and diltiazem. Unfortunately only about 10 to 15 percent of people with PPH will have a positive response, and only about 50 percent of them will have a long-term benefit from therapy with CCBs. Before the approval of new classes of agents, people with PPH were treated with CCBs, digitalis, diuretics, and blood thinners but these were often ineffective in improving symptoms or prolonging survival.

In the last few years, several new therapies have been developed for the treatment of PPH, but here we will discuss only those that can be taken orally or inhaled. (There is a chronic intravenous therapy for PPH.) These new therapies include *prostacyclin*-like medicines (also called *prostacyclin analogs*), *endothelin*, and *endothelin-receptor antagonists*, and *phosphodiesterase Type 5 inhibitors*. What these medicines have in common is that they all dilate the pulmonary arteries and arterioles.

PROSTACYCLIN ANALOGS

Prostacyclin belongs to a class of chemicals called *prostaglandins*. Prostaglandins were first discovered by a Swedish scientist named Ulf von Euler in the 1930s. He isolated a substance from semen that he thought came from the prostate, hence the name he gave it. Now we know that prostaglandins are chemical substances manufactured by almost every cell in the body. They have multiple actions and can either constrict or dilate blood vessels. A prostaglandin called *thromboxane* stimulates blood vessels to contract and prompts platelets to clump together, forming a clot. Prostaglandins can activate the inflammatory response. Other prostaglandins are involved in inducing labor in pregnant women (and other mammals).

There are also substances that break down or inhibit prostaglandin, both manufactured and naturally occurring. For example, aspirin is a prostaglandin inhibitor, which accounts for its favorable effect on inflammation and clotting. The *nonsteroidal anti-inflammatory drugs (NSAIDs)* are also prostaglandin inhibitors.

Prostacylin is a prostaglandin that dilates blood vessels. The intravenous form of prostacyclin, called *epoprostenol*, was the first drug that was proven to lower the risk of death in people with severe PPH, when it was given chronically.

Iloprost is an inhaled form of prostacyclin that not only dilates the pulmonary arteries, it also interferes with clotting, a feature of PPH. Iloprost is administered by inhalation in a dose of 2.5 to 5.0 mcg six to nine times daily, during waking hours, and not more than once every two hours.

The most common side effects among people taking iloprost are flushing, cough, headache, and nausea. Increased shortness of breath, chest pain, and supraventricular tachycardia also have been reported. When iloprost is used with other medicines that dilate blood vessels, abnormally low blood pressure can occur, and because iloprost interferes with clotting, people taking other blood thinners might be at increased risk of bleeding. However, because almost all people with PPH are on long-term blood thinners given the risk of clotting in this condition, this possible interaction is not considered to be clinically important.

An oral form of prostacyclin, called Beraprost, has been approved for use in PPH in Japan and South Korea but has not been approved by the FDA in the United States. The other prostacyclin-like medicine, *epoprostenol,* can only be administered intravenously, so will not be further discussed here.

ENDOTHELIN-RECEPTOR ANTAGONISTS

Endothelin (ET) is a substance that can be considered as the antiprostacyclin. It is composed of 21 amino acids (*amino acids* are the building blocks of proteins) and it is manufactured in the wall of arteries. It is a very potent constrictor of blood vessels and causes overgrowth of the smooth muscle cells in the media of arteries. Increased levels of ET in the blood and lung tissue have been found in people with PPH.

In order to be effective, ET must be taken up by *receptors*, which are proteins on the surface of cells that bind to specific molecules. A variety of ET-receptor antagonists have been manufactured of which two, bosentan and ambrisentan, have been approved by the FDA for use in people with moderate to severe PPH, defined as those who have symptoms with minimal exertion or at rest. This is the only use for which they been approved.

The first ET-receptor blocker to be approved by the FDA was bosentan. Bosentan's prescribing is very tightly controlled through the manufacturer's access program; you can't buy this drug in your local pharmacy. The reason for this is that bosentan can cause severe liver damage and birth defects. Women of childbearing age need to have a pregnancy test to be certain they are not pregnant before taking this drug and must use effective birth control. Monthly pregnancy tests are recommended for women on bosentan. In animal testing, bosentan often caused congenital defects.

Liver enzyme tests must be checked every month in people taking bosentan, and the drug must be discontinued if significant abnormalities occur. Bosentan should not be prescribed if liver bloods tests called aminotransferases are elevated three or more times the upper limit of normal. There are set protocols for stopping or decreasing the dose of bosentan based on the extent of aminotransferase elevations. Signs of liver injury, in addition to blood test results, include nausea, jaundice, fatigue, vomiting, malaise (feeling awful), unusual lethargy, fever, and abdominal pain. If these symptoms occur, or if another blood test of liver function (bilirubin) is elevated more than twice the upper limit of normal bosentan should be stopped.

Less-serious potential side effects include flushing, drop in blood pressure, swelling of the legs, palpitations, and itching. There also have been several cases of allergic reactions, manifested as angioedema in people taking bosentan.

Elevated blood levels of bosentan can occur in people who are taking certain other medicines that are metabolized by the liver, as bosentan is. These other medicines include ketoconazole, amiodarone, fluconazole, ritonavir, and itraconazole. Bosentan should not be used at the same time as these medicines. In addition, because of an increased risk of side effects, bosentan should not be used by people on the diabetic medicine glyburide, and by people who have had transplants and are taking cyclosporine. Bosentan was shown to lower the serum levels of hormones in women taking Ortho Novum at the same time. Therefore, ovulation may not be suppressed by hormonal birth control in women taking bosentan and pregnancy prevention in women on bosentan requires the use of additional barrier forms of contraception.

Bosentan lowers blood pressure in both the systemic (body) arteries and the pulmonary arteries. Along with this, the amount of blood ejected by the heart, what is called the *cardiac output*, increases. In studies of this medicine in people with PPH, bosentan has improved exercise ability, decreased shortness of breath, and decreased the need for hospitalizations. It is not known if survival is improved in people who take this medicine. Bosentan is taken in a dose of 62.5 mg to 125 mg twice a day.

In 2007, a second endothelin receptor antagonist, ambrisentan, was approved by the FDA for the treatment of PPH. Ambrisentan improves the ability of people with PPH to exercise and slows down the progressive worsening that is usually a feature of this disease. It appears to have less risk of liver damage than bosentan but the FDA still requires that doctors monitor patients on this drug each month with blood tests to look for liver damage. Headache is the most common side effect reported by people taking ambrisentan. Ambrisentan also can cause flushing, swelling of the feet and ankles, nasal congestion, and inflammation of the sinuses. It only needs to be taken once a day, unlike bosentan. Like bosentan, it is only available through a restricted distribution program

Ambrisentan does not appear to affect the activity or dosage of warfarin. It is contraindicated in pregnant women because of the risk of birth defects. People with moderate or severe liver disease cannot take this drug. The usual dose is 5 to 10 mg daily. Another endothelin receptor antagonist, sitaxentan, currently is awaiting FDA approval.

PHOSPHODIESTERASE TYPE 5 INHIBITORS

Phosphodiesterase inhibitors are a group of molecules that inhibit enzymes involved in chemical signaling within cells. *Phosphodiesterase 5 (PDE 5)* is one of more than 10 families of phosphodiesterases that have been discovered. PDE 5 is abundant in vascular smooth muscle, and inhibiting it leads to relaxation of smooth muscle and dilation of the blood vessel. PDE 5 inhibitors burst into public awareness on March 27, 1998, when the FDA approved the use of sildenafil (Viagra®) for erectile dysfunction, what used to be referred to as impotence. Suddenly, a topic that was rarely mentioned in polite society was all over the airwaves as spokesmen including the soccer star Pele, Texas Ranger hitter Rafael Palmeiro, and former Senate Majority leader and presidential candidate Bob Dole extolled Viagra's ability to enhance their sexual prowess. Pfizer, the drug company holding the patent, had a winner on its hands and doctors could hardly keep up with the demand for prescriptions.

It was not long after its approval by the FDA that studies were undertaken to see if sildenafil, given its ability to dilate blood vessels, might be useful in the treatment

Table 6–1 Drugs Used in the Treatment of Primary Pulmonary Hypertension

Drug (Trade) Name	Usual Daily Dose
Iloprost (Ventavis®)	2.5–5.0 mcg (inhaled 6–9 times/day while awake)
Bosentan (Tracleer®)	125–250 mg/d
Ambrisentan (Letairis®)	5–10 mg/d
Sildenafil (Revatio®)	60 mg/d

of PPH. These controlled trials showed that sildenafil causes an increase in exercise ability and cardiac output and a decrease in pulmonary artery pressures in people with PPH.

Sildenafil when used to treat PPH is marketed under a different name (Revatio®) and unlike Viagra®, which is taken as needed in a dose of 50 or 100 mg, Revatio is taken on a daily basis in a dose of 20 mg three times a day to treat PPH. Potential side effects of the two preparations are the same. They include headache, flushing, upset stomach, color perception distortion, nosebleeds, insomnia, diarrhea, and a drop in blood pressure that may be enough to cause dizziness. Sildenafil should not be taken with itraconazole, ketoconazole, or ritonavir. Because of the risk of a severe drop in blood pressure, nitrate medicines and alpha-blocking medicines should not be taken by people who are on sildenafil. More recently, the occurrence of sudden visual loss, which may be temporary or permanent, has been reported in men taking PDE 5 inhibitors for erectile dysfunction. Most of these men have had other risk factors for developing the specific eye problem, called *nonarteritic anterior ischemic optic neuropathy (NAION)*, responsible for the vision loss, such as smoking, diabetes, coronary artery disease, age over 50, hypertension, and hyperlipidemia.

On Oct. 18, 2007 the FDA issued an alert about sildenafil (and the other medicines in this class) warning of the potential for sudden hearing loss, ringing in the ears and dizziness, requiring more prominent display of these risks. Because Revatio is used to treat a potentially life-threatening condition, the FDA did not recommend that patients abruptly stop taking this medication but advised them to contact their physician if they experience sudden problems with their hearing.

In animal studies, sildenafil, unlike bosentan, did not cause congenital defects, but its safety in human pregnancy has not been established. It is unknown if sildenafil is excreted in breast milk. Another PDE 5 inhibitor, tadalafil (Cialis®), currently is being studied to see if it is effective in the treatment of PPH.

Table 6–1 lists the drugs currently available to treat PPH. These are usually added to a regimen that includes digoxin, diuretics, CCBs, and the blood thinner warfarin.

CHAPTER 7

Anticoagulant and Anti-Platelet Agents: The Blood Thinners

ASPIRIN

Anticoagulants and anti-platelet agents are medicines that make the blood less likely to clot. They are referred to as "blood thinners" but they don't actually thin the blood. The different medicines that interfere with the formation of clots can all increase the risk of bleeding or hemorrhage. The most commonly prescribed of these medicines is aspirin, and even though it can be obtained without a prescription it is important for anyone with cardiovascular disease to be aware of the benefits and risks of this useful drug.

Clots are involved in most acute cardiovascular events such as heart attacks and strokes, so medicines to inhibit the formation of clots play a large role in the treatment (and even the prevention) of cardiovascular disease. The oldest such medicine, is aspirin, the name given by the German pharmaceutical company Friedrich Bayer & Co. to a new drug it patented in 1899.

The chemical name for aspirin is *acetylsalicylic acid (ASA)*. Dr. Felix Hoffman, a chemist employed by Friedrich Bayer & Company, was one of the first to synthesize ASA. It was originally used to treat pain, inflammation, and fever.

However, the therapeutic effects of a similar compound were known for thousands of years before Hoffman's work. Hippocrates, considered the father of scientific medicine and the most famous physician in ancient Greece, prescribed an extract of willow tree bark to treat pain and fever more than 2500 years ago. Native Americans also used extracts of tree barks to treat various disorders, and willow extracts were well known for their effect on pain and fever in Europe for centuries. The active ingredient in these concoctions is salicin, which is converted in the body to salicylic acid. It was first isolated by chemists in both France and Italy in 1828. Salicylic acid proved to be very irritating to the stomach and by modifying the structure of salicylic acid and producing acetylsalicylic acid, Dr. Hoffman was able to make a medicine that was effective and had fewer side effects.

The mechanism by which aspirin exerted its beneficial effects was not known until 1971, when a British pharmacologist, John Vane, showed that aspirin inhibited the production of prostaglandins. (See Chapter 6 for a discussion of prostaglandins.) Dr. Vane received a knighthood and the Nobel Prize for his work.

It is aspirin's effect in opposing the action of the prostaglandin thromboxane that is responsible for its effect on inhibiting the formation of clots. Aspirin prevents the clumping together of platelets, which are crucial to clot formation. This effect occurs within minutes of aspirin being absorbed into the bloodstream and lasts for 4 to 7 days. Aspirin is absorbed rapidly when it is taken by mouth. The dose of aspirin needed to inhibit clotting is much less than the dose needed to treat fever and inflammation. As little as 81 mg of aspirin every other day will lower the risk of clots; doses of 1000 to 5000 mg a day are used to treat inflammation.

Despite the fact that aspirin is a nonprescription drug, it has a significant risk of side effects. The most common of these is stomach irritation, at times leading to bleeding into the gastrointestinal (GI) tract. The amount of blood loss caused by aspirin is increased at higher doses but even at low doses, aspirin increases the risk of GI bleeding. At higher doses, aspirin can cause ringing in the ears, vomiting, vertigo, and decreased hearing. Liver function test abnormalities can occur from aspirin but these tend to be mild. People with chronic liver disease in general should not take aspirin. Women should avoid taking aspirin in the last third of pregnancy because it increases the risk of bleeding during labor and delivery. An allergy to aspirin can develop in susceptible people. This is most frequently manifested as an itchy rash called *urticaria* or *hives*.

Hemophiliacs, because of the increased risk of bleeding, should not take aspirin. People who are allergic to aspirin must avoid it and any combination painkiller that contains aspirin. People who are taking warfarin have an increased risk of bleeding while on aspirin, but there are certain cardiac patients in whom the benefits of taking both warfarin and aspirin outweigh the risks, such as those with artificial heart valves. The combination of aspirin and another blood thinner, clopidogrel, increases the risk of bleeding but is used routinely in people who have stents put into their arteries to keep them open, where again, the benefit has been proven to outweigh the risk.

Aspirin can lower the risk of heart attack when taken prophylactically by healthy men. However, the Women's Health Aspirin study of more than 27,000 healthy women aged 45 or older who took 100 mg of aspirin every other day showed that in women, although aspirin lowered the risk of stroke by 17 percent when compared to a placebo, there was no decrease in the risk of heart attack. When the study data were reanalyzed looking only at women who were 65 or older at entry into the study, it was found that healthy older women who took aspirin lowered their risk of stroke by 30 percent and heart attack by 34 percent, compared to women who took the placebo. Both men and women who have established vascular disease lower their risk of future events when they take low-dose aspirin, so unless there is a very strong contraindication, all people with vascular disease should take aspirin.

WARFARIN

Rodenticide is a fancy term for rat killer and that's the first use warfarin was put to. Rats and their fellow travelers, particularly fleas, have a long fascinating connection with humans in the annals of the history of medicine. The best known example of a rat/flea–borne illness is the Black Death (also called the Black Plague or bubonic plague), an epidemic that decimated the populations of Asia and Europe in the 14th century. It recurred often over the next few centuries but since the 18th century, it has only occurred sporadically, not in epidemic form.

The bacteria thought to have caused this illness, *yersinia pestis*, was not discovered until 1894 and the people in the countries afflicted by plague devised fanciful explanations for the dread disease which, in some areas carried off two-thirds of the population. Most of these explanations centered around perceived divine punishment for man's sins or the deliberate poisoning of wells by Jews. Scores of Jewish communities were destroyed and so-called *flagellant societies* arose, whose members flogged themselves to atone for their sins. However, nothing seemed to lessen the toll of this dread disease. Belief in the Catholic church waned and disillusionment with its clergy, who were helpless to halt the spread of the plague, became widespread. With the precipitous drop in population, the economy of Europe was plunged into a recession that lasted for decades.

Salmonella, typhus, rabies, and leptospirosis are some of the many other diseases that can be caused by exposure to rats or the insects they host.

Long before researchers knew about the connection between rats and human disease, they were already hated for their theft of precious food stores. Rats are avid consumers of crops and destroy property by gnawing. Today, it is estimated that about a quarter of electrical cable breakage is caused by rats. For centuries, people kept pets specifically for their ability to catch and eat rats. Cats, snakes, and specially bred dogs (for instance, rat terriers) are the commonest examples. Human rat catchers often were hired by towns to rid themselves of severe infestations—remember the old story "The Pied Piper"?

The breed called rat terriers was developed in Britain in 1820 and imported into the United States in 1890. They were derived from Manchester Terriers and Smooth Fox Terriers, and President Teddy Roosevelt was an early fan of the breed. Yorkshire terriers were used by weavers in 19th century to guard their products from being eaten by rats.

The poisoning of rats has a long history. Cyanide, strychnine, and arsenic were among the chemicals used in the past to kill rats. However, the extreme danger of these poisons to humans made their widespread use problematic. Warfarin was developed originally as a rat poison in 1948. It was derived from a naturally occurring plant molecule called *coumarin*. The clot-inhibiting action of coumarin was discovered in the 1930s when cows who had eaten spoilt clover died of hemorrhage. In 1939, the agent that caused the hemorrhage was isolated and named *bishydroxycoumarin* or *coumarin*. However, fear of its danger kept it from being used as a clot inhibitor in humans until 1951 when an Army inductee tried to commit suicide by taking a massive overdose of warfarin, but survived. Since then, warfarin has been used extensively in various cardiovascular conditions and has saved many lives.

Warfarin works by blocking the synthesis of certain clotting factors, those dependent on the action of vitamin K, and the synthesis of two other anticlotting blood proteins called protein C and protein S. Vitamin K is a fat-soluble vitamin that is found in various foods. It also is produced by bacteria in the bowel.

In order for blood to clot, for example, in response to a cut or an abnormality of a blood vessel wall (such as an artery with an unstable plaque), a very complex series of chemical reactions occurs, involving protein molecules called factors I thru XIII and the Von Willebrand factor. (The series of reactions that occurs in response to injury inside a blood vessel is referred to as the *intrinsic pathway*. The clotting that occurs in response to an external injury like a cut is called the *extrinsic pathway*.)

Platelets are microscopic formed elements in the blood that must form a clump and then be bound in a fibrin mesh in order for a stable clot to form. Think of fibrin as the glue that makes the platelets hang together. Clotting factor II is called prothrombin. Factor Xa activates prothrombin to form thrombin and thrombin in turn converts the inactive fibrinogen precursor into fibrin.

The clotting factors that depend on the presence of vitamin K are factors II, VII, IX, and X. It takes three to four days for the effect of warfarin to be measurable and the amount of interference with clotting is monitored by a blood test called a *prothrombin time (PT)* or *international normalized ratio (INR)*. PT is the amount of time in seconds that it takes for blood plasma to clot after being exposed to tissue factor (factor III). The INR takes into account differences in strength between various batches of tissue factor. It is a ratio between the measured PT and the PT of a normal sample raised to the power of an *international sensitivity index (ISI)*. (The ISI is a value that each manufacturer of tissue factor gives to each batch they produce.) The normal range for PT is approximately 12 to 15 seconds and for INR is 0.8 to 1.2.

If someone has to take warfarin because they have developed a clot in the heart, in the deep veins of the leg, or are in atrial fibrillation, the INR will be regulated at values between 2.0 and 3.0. If someone has an artificial heart valve, their INR will be regulated between values of 2.5 and 3.5. Particularly in people who have artificial heart valves, a low dose of aspirin often is prescribed in addition to warfarin.

People may require doses of warfarin between 1 and 10 mg a day to achieve these INR levels. Especially when someone first starts taking warfarin, frequent blood tests are required before that individual's proper dose of warfarin can be determined. More importantly, even people who have had a stable INR for many months may require either a higher or lower warfarin dose if they develop an acute illness or another medicine is added to their regimen.

For example, if a person on warfarin develops diarrhea and stops eating, he or she will take in less vitamin K and their INR may become very prolonged, leading to bleeding—or, because vitamin K is made by bacteria in the bowel, people on antibiotics that kill these bacteria may develop very low levels of vitamin K, and a previously therapeutic dose of warfarin will lead to a marked prolongation of the PT/INR, with increased risk of bleeding.

People who start taking warfarin often are told to avoid green, leafy vegetables, because they are rich in vitamin K, however, these vegetables are part of a heart-healthy diet. I tell my patients to continue eating vitamin K–rich foods, but to keep the intake of these foods stable. The warfarin dose can be adjusted to account for this. In addition to green leafy vegetables, other vitamin K–rich foods include liver, cauliflower, green tea, chick peas, cheese, alfalfa sprouts, beef, pork, whole milk, strawberries, oats, extra virgin olive oil, canola oil, and cottonseed oil.

Another potential problem for people on warfarin is the taking of nonprescription herbal remedies. Some herbal products can block the action of warfarin, increasing the risk of clots, and others may enhance its action, increasing the risk of bleeding. It is vital that your physician knows every medicine, whether prescription or nonprescription, that you are taking while on warfarin.

Because vitamin K is fat soluble, people unable to absorb fat from the diet (called malabsorption) may develop vitamin K deficiency. People with chronic liver disease can have vitamin K deficiency, as can people on chronic antibiotic therapy. People with vitamin K deficiency may have a prolonged INR, even if they are not taking warfarin, so if such people need to take warfarin, they are likely to need a lower dose to achieve a therapeutic INR. In the presence of severe liver disease, the liver may be unable to make the clotting factors needed for normal blood coagulation. In that situation, the INR may be prolonged even in people not taking warfarin, so treating such a patient with warfarin would be dangerous. People with severe kidney disease who require warfarin also must be monitored very carefully. People over the age of 60 are more sensitive to the effect of warfarin and usually require a lower dose to achieve a therapeutic INR than younger people. People of Asian descent also seem to be more sensitive to warfarin.

The most common side effect of warfarin, not surprisingly, is easy bruising; a more serious side effect is bleeding. This can occur spontaneously even if the INR is not prolonged outside of the therapeutic range. However, if the INR is in the therapeutic range and bleeding occurs, it is often because there is a previously unknown abnormality, such as an ulcer or polyp. More than a few people have had a malignancy diagnosed when they are treated with warfarin and, for example, their cancerous colon polyp suddenly starts to bleed.

Another potential serious side effect of warfarin is embolization of particles called *cholesterol emboli*. (*Embolization* is the process by which an organ or blood vessel is obstructed by material; in this case, plaque material containing cholesterol and clot that travels there from someplace else.) Embolization of this material, depending on where it lodges, can lead to kidney failure, stroke, pancreatic inflammation, gangrene of the skin or limbs, and even death.

There are literally dozens of medications that can either enhance the effect of warfarin or block the effect of warfarin. If you need to start one of these medicines, your INR will need to be checked more frequently and your doctor may either increase or decrease your dose of warfarin. The medicines that may enhance the effect of warfarin are listed in Table 7–1. Medicines that have been reported to decrease the effect of warfarin can be found in Table 7–2. To make matters more

Table 7–1 Medicines Reported to Increase the Effect of Warfarin

Allopurinol (Zyloprim®)	Itraconazole (Sporanox®)	Piroxicam (Feldene®)
Aspirin (Ecotrin, Bayer ASA)	Ketoprofen (Orudis®)	Propafenone (Rythmol®)
	Ketorolac (Toradol®)	Propoxyphene (Darvon®)
Amiodarone (Cordarone®)	Lansoprazole (Prevacid®)	Propanolol (Inderal®)
Azithromycin (Zithromax®)	Levamisole (Ergamisol®)	Quinidine (Quinaglute®)
Capecitabine (Xeloda®)	Levofloxacin (Levaquin®)	Quinine (Quinine S04®)
Celecoxib (Celebrex®)	Levothyroxine	Rabeprazole (Aciphex®)
Cimetidine (Tagamet®)	(Synthroid®, Levoxyl®,	Sertraline (Zoloft®)
Ciprofloxacin (Cipro®)	Unithroid®)	Simvastatin (Zocor®)
Clarithromycin (Biaxin®)	Lovastatin (Mevacor®,	Stanozolol (Winstrol®)
Clofibrate (Atromid-S®)	Altoprev®)	Sulfamethoxazole
Danazol (Danocrine®)	Mefenamic (Ponstel®)	(Gantanol®)
Diclofenac (Voltaren®)	Methylphenidate (Ritalin®)	Sulfisoxazole (Gantrisin®)
Diflunisal (Dolobid®)	Metronidazole (Flagyl®)	Sulindac (Clinoril®)
Disulfiram (Antabuse®)	Nalidixic acid (Neggram®)	Tamoxifen (Nolvadex®)
Doxycycline (Monodox®)	Naproxen (Naprosyn®)	Tetracycline (Sumycin®)
Erythromycin	Neomycin	Ticlopidine (Ticlid®)
(Erythrocin®)	Norfloxacin (Noroxin®)	Tramadol (Ultram®)
Esomeprazole (Nexium®)	Ofloxacin (Floxin®)	Trimethoprim/Sulfametho
Fenofibrate (Tricor®)	Olsalazine (Dipentum®)	xazole (Bactrim®,
Fenoprofen (Nalfon®)	Omeprazole (Prilosec®)	Bactrim DS®)
Fluconazole (Diflucan®)	Oxandrolone (Oxandrin®)	Ticlopidine (Ticlid®)
Fluoxetine (Prozac®)	Oxaprozin (Daypro®)	Tramadol (Ultram®)
Flutamide (Eulexin®)	Oxymetholone	Valdecoxib (Bextra®)
Fluvastatin (Lescol®)	(Anadrol-50®)	Valproate (Depakote®)
Fluvoxamine (Luvox®)	Pantoprazole (Protonix®)	Vitamin E
Gefitinib (Iressa®)	Paroxetine (Asimia®)	Zafirlukast (Accolate®)
Gemfibrozil (Lopid®)	Pentoxifylline (Trental®)	Zileuton (Zyflo®)
Ibuprofen (Motrin, Advil)	Phenylbutazone	
Indomethacin (Indocin®)	(Butazolidine®)	

Table 7–2 Medicines That Have Been Reported to Decrease the Effect of Warfarin

Aminoglutethimide (Cytadren®)   Raloxifene (Evista®)
Carbamazepine (Tegretol®)   Rifampin (Rifadin®)
Griseofulvin (Fulvicin®)   Sucralfate (Carafate®)
Pentobarbital (Nembutal®)

Table 7–3 Medicines Reported to Both Increase and Decrease the Effect of Warfarin

Chloral hydrate (Noctec®)   Phenytoin (Dilantin®)
Cholestyramine (Questran®)   Prednisone (Deltasone®)
Cortisone (Cortone®)   Propylthiouracil
Cyclophosphamide   Ranitidine (Zantac®)
Methimazole (Tapazole®)   Trazadone (Desyrel®)

---

complicated, there are some medicines that have been reported to both increase and decrease the effect of warfarin. Table 7–3 displays these.

Despite the risk of serious side effects, many scientifically valid studies have shown that warfarin treatment lowers the risk of stroke in people who have AF and artificial heart valves. Warfarin also lowers the risk that an artificial heart valve will become obstructed by clots, which can lead to severe heart failure and even death.

The use of warfarin in pregnant women with artificial heart valves is contraindicated because there is a risk of congenital abnormalities and an increased risk of miscarriage. In this situation, another blood thinner that only can be taken by injection is used. Nursing mothers, however, can take warfarin without affecting their baby's blood's ability to clot.

On August 16, 2007, the FDA updated the label for warfarin to include information about new genetic testing that might identify people who could be more susceptible to adverse effects. Genetic variants of two different genes are thought to cause about 35 to 50 percent of the variability in dose response to warfarin, and people with these genes may require a lower initial dose of the drug (see Table 7–4). However, no studies have been done to show that using these genetic tests has an impact on the safety of warfarin. Table 7–4 lists the oral anticoagulant warfarin and its usual daily dose.

PLATELET INHIBITORS

Clopidogrel is another blood-thinning medicine, which, like aspirin, helps prevent platelets from clumping together and forming a clot. It blocks a receptor on the surface of platelets that helps fibrin bind the platelets together. It is used extensively

Table 7–4 Oral Anticoagulant (Blood Thinner)

Drug (Trade) Name	Dosage Range (mg/d)
Warfarin (Coumadin®)	1–10 mg

in people with coronary artery disease, peripheral vascular disease, and cerebrovascular disease. It may be used instead of aspirin in people who have aspirin allergy, but often is used in conjunction with aspirin; for example, in people who have had stents placed in their arteries. Clopidogrel sometimes is given to people who are having an acute coronary syndrome, especially when a stent procedure is planned. A loading dose of 150 to 300 mg is given in that situation, followed by a daily dose of 75 mg. Clopidogrel must be taken with aspirin for at least a year by people who have had a drug-coated stent placed in a coronary artery. Clopidogrel and aspirin also are used together in peripheral arterial disease and in people who have carotid artery disease.

The most common side effect of clopidogrel is bruising and the most significant is bleeding which can occur into the stomach, bowel, bladder, or in response to trauma. It is much less likely to cause a fall in white blood cells or a rare condition called TTP than is ticlodipine (see the following section).

Ticlopidine

Ticlopidine is another medicine in this class of platelet inhibitors. It blocks the same platelet receptor that clopidogrel does. It was approved by the FDA before clopidogrel but has a side effect that clopidogrel doesn't: In some people, it causes a drop in the white blood cell count, which can be severe enough to increase the risk of infection. Rarely, ticlopidine can also cause a serious illness called *thrombotic thrombocytopenic purpura (TTP)*, which can lead to kidney failure and can cause the bone marrow to stop making red blood cells, a condition called *aplastic anemia*. For this reason, people taking ticlopidine must have regular blood tests to look for these side effects. Nausea, vomiting, and diarrhea also can occur in people on this drug.

Despite these rare side effects, ticlopidine has been shown to be beneficial in people who have had strokes, or warning signs of stroke, when compared to aspirin, and in patients who have stents placed in a coronary artery. In both these situations, ticlopidine is used in conjunction with aspirin. The usual dose is 250 mg taken twice daily.

Dipyridamole

Dipyridamole is a mild platelet inhibitor and vasodilator that has no benefit as a clot preventer when used alone, but in combination with warfarin has been shown

Table 7–5 Platelet Inhibitors

Drug (Trade) Name	Usual Dose (mg/d)
Clopidogrel (Plavix®)	75
Ticlopidine (Ticlid®)	500
Dipyridamole (Persantine®)	300–400
Dipyridamole/aspirin (Aggrenox®)	400/50

to reduce the risk of clots forming and breaking off from artificial heart valves. There also is evidence from one study that taking dipyridamole with aspirin reduces the risk of stroke in people who have had a prior stroke or warning signs of a stroke. However, the only recommended use of dipyridamole at present is in combination with warfarin to prevent emboli in people with artificial heart valves. In that situation, it usually is taken in a dose of 75 to 100 mg four times daily. Dizziness, abdominal distress, and headache are the most frequently reported side effects of dipyridamole. Table 7–5 lists the commonly prescribed platelet inhibitors or combinations and their usual daily doses.

With judicious use of these clot inhibitors, the risks of atherosclerotic cardiovascular disease complications such as heart attacks and strokes can be lowered, in many cases dramatically.

Readings

A-HeFT.org. African American Heart Failure Test. Available at: www.aheft.org/about.asp. Accessed November 8, 2007.

American Heart Association. Angina pectoris. Available at: www.americanheart.org/presenter.jhtml?identifier=4472. Accessed November 21, 2007.

American Heart Association. Atrial fibrillation. Available at: www.americanheart.org/presenter.jhtml?identifier=4451. Accessed November 12, 2007.

American Heart Association and American Stroke Association. Heart disease and stroke Statistics. Available at: www.americanheart.org/downloadable/heart/1166711577754HS_StatsInsideText.pdf. Accessed November 12, 2007.

Anderson J, Young L, Long E. Diet and hypertension. Colorado State University Extension. Available at: www.ext.colostate.edu/pubs/foodnut/09318.html. Accessed November 15, 2007.

Atrial Fibrillation Foundation. Common Q&A. 2005. Available at: www.affacts.org/Questions/torsades.html. Accessed November 9, 2007.

Atrial Fibrilation Foundation. Medications. 2005. Available at: www.affacts.org/Medications/medication_index.html. Accessed November 9, 2007.

Baker L. Research links cholesterol, hypertension. *State University of New York at Buffalo Reporter*. 1997, July 24. Available at: www.buffalo.edu/reporter/vol28/vol28n35/f2.html. Accessed November 13, 2007.

Battegay E, Bakris GL, Lip GYH, eds. *Hypertension: Principles and Practice*. Boca Raton, FL: Taylor & Francis Group, LLC;2005.

Black HR, ed. *Clinical Trials in Hypertension*. New York: Marcel Dekker, Inc.; 2001.

Braunwald E. Heart failure and corpulmonale. In DL Kasper, E Braunwald, AS Fauci, SL Hauser, DL Longo, & JL Jameson, eds. *Harrison's Principles of Internal Medicine*. New York: McGraw-Hill.

Carson PE, Johnson GR, Dunkman WB, Fletcher RD, Farrell L, Cohn JN. The influence of atrial fibrillation on prognosis in mild to moderate heart failure. The V-HeFT Studies. *Circulation*. 1993; 87(6 Suppl):VI102–1110.

Digitalis Investigation Group. The effect of digoxin on mortality and morbidity in patients with heart failure. *New England Journal of Medicine*. 1997;336(8): 525–533.

Felmeden D, Nadar SK, Lip GYH. Aspirin and endothelial function in hypertension. *Journal of Human Hypertension*. 2005;19:663–665.

The Franklin Institute. Healthy hearts: Hypertension. Available at: www.fi.edu/learn/heart/healthy/pressure.html. Accessed November 14, 2007.

Harris WS, Appel LJ. New guidelines focus on fish, fish oil, omega-3 fatty acids. 2002. Available at: www.americanheart.org/presenter.jhtml?identifier=3006624. Accessed November 8, 2007.

Heart Rhythm Society. Atrial fibrillation facts. Available at: www.hrsonline.org/News/Media/fact-sheets/Atrial-Fibrillation-Facts.cfm. Accessed November 9, 2007.

86   Readings

Herrick JB. Clinical features of sudden obstruction of the coronary arteries. *Journal of the American Medical Association.* 1912;59:2015–2019.

Hurst W. *The Heart, Arteries, and Veins.* 10th ed. New York: McGraw-Hill; 2002.

International Society on Hypertension in Blacks. About hypertension. 2005. Available at: www.ishib.org/HI_abohyp.asp. Accessed October 31, 2007.

Jackson G. *Hypertension in Women.* London: Martin Dunitz, Ltd.; 1996.

Jeffrey D. *Aspirin: The Remarkable Story of a Wonder Drug.* New York: Bloomsbury; 2004.

Katz AM. *Physiology of the Heart.* 4th ed. Philadelphia: Lippincott Williams & Wilkins; 2005.

Kulick D. Congestive heart failure. Available at: www.medicinenet.com/congestive_heart_failure/article.htm. Accessed November 7, 2007.

Lipsky MS, Mendelson M, Havas S, Miller M. *American Medical Association Guide to Preventing and Treating Heart Disease: Essential Information You and Your Family Need to Know About Having a Healthy Heart.* Hoboken, NJ: John Wiley and Sons, Inc.; 2008.

Mayo Clinic. Statins: Are these cholesterol-lowering drugs right for you? 2006. Available at: www.mayoclinic.com/health/statins/CL00010. Accessed November 16, 2007.

Mayo Foundation for Medical Education and Research. 2006. Angiotensin II receptor blockers. Available at: www.mayoclinic.com/health/angiotensin-II-receptor-blockers/HI00054. Accessed November 20, 2007.

MedlinePlus. Warfarin. Available at: www.nlm.nih.gov/medlineplus/druginfo/medmaster/a682277.html. Accessed November 22, 2007.

Murrell W. Nitro-glycerin as a remedy for angina pectoris. *Lancet.*1879;80:113_115.

National Heart, Lung, and Blood Institute. The Seventh Report of the Joint National Committee on Prevention, Detection, Evaluation, and Treatment of High Blood Pressure. 2004. Available at: www.nhlbi.nih.gov/guidelines/hypertension/. Accessed November 23, 2007.

National Heart, Lung, and Blood Institute. *The Framingham Study: An Epidemiological Investigation of Cardiovascular Disease.* Washington, DC: U.S.Government Printing Office; 1973. Available at: www.framinghamheartstudy.org.

The Nobel Foundation. Nobel prizes: John R. Vane. Available at: http://nobelprize.org/nobel_prizes/medicine/laureates/1982/vane-autobio.html. Accessed November 22, 2007.

Oliver JJ, Melville VP, Webb DJ. Effect of regular phosphodiesterase type 5 inhibition in hypertension. *Hypertension.* 2006; 48:622–627.

Pfizer, Inc.Viagra. Available at: www.viagra.com/content/index.jsp?setShowOn=../content/index.jsp&setShowHighlightOn=../content/index.jsp. Accessed November 13, 2007.

Pitt B, Remme W, Zannad F, et al. Eplerenone, a selective aldosterone blocker, in patients with left ventricular dysfunction after myocardial infarction. *New England Journal of Medicine.* 2003; 348(22):2271.

Pitt B, Zannad F, Remme W, et al. The effect of spironolactone on morbidity and mortality in patients with severe heart failure. *New England Journal of Medicine.* 1999;341:709–717.

Poole-Wilson PA, Swedberg K, Cleland JGF, et al. COMET investigators comparison of carvedilol and metoprolol on clinical outcomes in patients with chronic heart failure in the Carvedilol Or Metoprolol European Trial (COMET) randomised controlled trial. *Lancet.* 2003;362:7–13.

Pulmonary Hypertension Association. What is PH?Available at: www.phassociation.org/Learn/What-is-PH/index.asp. Accessed November 26, 2007.

Ridker PM, Cook NR, Lee I-M, et al. A randomized trial of low-dose aspirin in the primary prevention of cardiovascular disease in women. *New England Journal of Medicine.* 2005;352(13):1293–1304.

Shekelle PG, Rich MW, Morton SC, et al. Efficacy of angiotensin-converting enzyme inhibitors and beta-blockers in the management of left ventricular systolic dysfunction according to race, gender, and diabetic status. *Journal of the American College of Cardiology.* 2003;41:1529–1538.

Shopland D, ed. Risks associated with smoking cigarettes with low machine-measured yields of tar and nicotine. *Smoking and Tobacco Control*. 2001. Available at: http://cancercontrol.cancer.gov/tcrb/monographs/13/m13_complete.pdf. Accessed October 31, 2007.

Szromba C. ACE inhibitors and ARBs: Antihypertensive medications in CKD. *Nephrology Nursing Journal*. 2005;32(3):332–333.

Taber CL Taber's Cyclopedic Medical Dictionary. Philadelphia: F.A. Davis Co., 1964.

U.S. Dept. of Health and Human Services. Available at http://cancercontrol.cancer.gov/tcrb/monographs/13/m13_complete.pdf. Accessed Jan 21, 2008.

U.S. Food and Drug Administration. FDA approves new orphan drug for treatment of pulmonary arterial hypertension. Available at: www.fda.gov/bbs/topics/NEWS/2007/NEW01653.html. Accessed November 14, 2007.

U.S. Food and Drug Administration. Questions and answers on new labeling for warfarin. Available at: www.fda.gov/cder/drug/infopage/warfarin/qa.htm. Accessed November 14, 2007.

U.S. Food and Drug Administration. Viagra (sildenafil citrate) information. Available at: www.fda.gov/cder/consumerinfo/viagra/default.htm. Accessed November 23, 2007.

U.S. Food and Drug Administration, Center for Drug Evaluation and Research.Fen-Phen information. 2001. Available at: www.fda.gov/cder/news/feninfo.htm. Accessed November 26, 2007.

U.S. Food and Drug Administration, Center for Drug Evaluation and Research. 1998. Drug approvals for March 1998. www.fda.gov/cder/da/da0398.htm. Accessed November 14, 2007.

U.S. National Library of Medicine & National Institutes of Health. Wolff-Parkinson-White syndrome. 2006. Available at: www.nlm.nih.gov/medlineplus/ency/article/000151.htm#Definition. Accessed November 22, 2007.

Venes D. *Taber's Cyclopedic Medical Dictionary*. Philadelphia: F.A. Davis Company; 2005.

von Euler U. *Prostaglandins*. London: Academic Press; 1967.

Westmaas JL, Nath V, Brandon TH. Contemporary smoking cessation. 2000. *Journal of the Moffitt Cancer Center*. Available at: www.moffitt.org/moffittapps/ccj//v7n1/article5.htm. Accessed October 31, 2007.

Withering W. *An Account of the Foxglove and Some of Its Medical Uses*. London: The Broomsleigh Press; 1785.

Zipes DP, Libby P, Bonow R, Braunwald E, eds. *Braunwald's Heart Disease: A Textbook of Cardiovascular Medicine*. 7th ed. Philadelphia: Saunders; 2004.

Glossary

Ablation: The process of destroying tissue; for example, ablation may be used to destroy an area in the heart that is causing an abnormal heart rhythm.

Acebutolol: A beta-blocker used to treat high blood pressure; also called Sectral®.

Aldosterone: A substance released by the adrenal glands that causes the body to retain potassium and excrete sodium.

Aliskiren: A direct renin inhibitor; used to treat high blood pressure; also called Tekturna®.

Ambrisentan: A medicine used to treat primary pulmonary hypertension; also called Letairis®.

Amiloride: A diuretic used in the treatment of high blood pressure; also called Midamor®.

Amiodarone: A medicine used in the treatment of abnormal heart rhythms; also called Cordarone® or Pacerone®.

Amlodipine: A calcium channel blocker used to treat high blood pressure and angina; also called Norvasc®.

Angina pectoris: A symptom that often occurs when the heart muscle is starved for oxygen; usually felt as a squeezing, burning, or pressing discomfort in the chest or elsewhere in the upper body; it is usually brought on by exertion or stress and goes away in a few minutes with nitroglycerin, rest, or relaxation.

Angiotensin receptor blocker (ARB): A class of medicines used to treat high blood pressure and congestive heart failure.

Angiotensin-converting enzyme inhibitor (ACE inhibitor): A class of medicines used to treat high blood pressure and congestive heart failure.

Anticoagulant: A medicine that makes the blood less likely to clot.

Arrhythmia: An abnormality of the heart rhythm.

Arteriosclerosis: Hardening of the arteries.

Artery: A blood vessel that carries oxygenated blood.

Aspirin: A commonly prescribed blood thinner.

Atenolol: A medicine used to treat angina and high blood pressure; also called Tenormin®.

Atherosclerosis: A form of arteriosclerosis in which plaque deposits build up in arteries.

Atherosclerotic cardiovascular disease (ASCVD): A disease of the heart and arteries caused by the build-up of plaque; the most common form of heart disease in the world.

Atorvastatin: A medicine used to treat high cholesterol; also called Lipitor®.

Atrial fibrillation: An arrhythmia in which the atria beat very fast and irregularly, causing the pulse to be rapid and irregular; it increases the risk of stroke.

Atrium (*pl.***atria**): The upper, receiving chambers of the heart.

Automatic implantable cardiac defibrillator (AICD) or **Implantable cardiac defibrillator (ICD):** A device that is inserted in the chest (usually through a vein) into the right side of the heart; it detects certain abnormal heart rhythms and delivers a shock to the heart to stop the arrhythmia.

Benazepril: An angiotensin-converting enzyme inhibitor (ACE) used in the treatment of high blood pressure; also called Lotensin®.

Bendroflumethazide: A diuretic used to treat high blood pressure; also called Naturetin®.

Beta-blocker: A class of medicines used to treat angina, high blood pressure, and sometimes, abnormal heart rhythms.

Betaxolol: A beta-blocker used to treat angina and high blood pressure; also called Kerlone®.

Bile acid sequestrants: A class of medicines that binds to bile in the intestines.

Bisoprolol: A beta-blocker used to treat angina, congestive heart failure, and high blood pressure; also called Zebeta®.

Bosentan: A medicine used to treat primary pulmonary hypertension; also called Tracleer®.

Bradycardia: An abnormal heart rhythm in which the heart beats too slowly; also called *bradyarrhythmia.*

Bumetanide: A diuretic used to treat high blood pressure and congestive heart failure; also called Bumex®.

Bupropion: A medicine used to treat nicotine addiction; also called Zyban®.

Calcium channel blocker (CCB): A class of medicines used to treat angina, high blood pressure, and sometimes, abnormal heart rhythms.

Candesartan: An angiotensin receptor blocker used to treat high blood pressure and congestive heart failure; also called Atacand®.

Capillaries: The smallest blood vessels; they can only be seen with a microscope; the blood vessels from which oxygen is given up by the blood to the tissues.

Captopril: An ACE inhibitor used in the treatment of high blood pressure and congestive heart failure; also called Capoten®.

Cardiomyopathy: Weakness of the heart muscle.

Cardiovascular: Relating to the heart and blood vessels.

Cardioversion: A procedure in which an electric shock is delivered to the heart, usually through the chest wall, to end an abnormal heart rhythm.

Carvedilol: A beta-blocker used to treat high blood pressure and congestive heart failure; also called Coreg® or Coreg CR®.

Chlorothiazide: A diuretic used to treat high blood pressure; also called Diuril®.

Chlorthalidone: A diuretic used to treat high blood pressure; also called Hygroton®.

Cholesterol: A waxy substance found in every cell of the body that is important in the manufacture of many hormones; high levels of cholesterol increase the risk of atherosclerosis.

Cholestyramine: A bile acid sequestrant used to treat high blood levels of cholesterol; also called Questran®.

Chylomicron: Blood fat formed from dietary fat; very-high levels can cause attacks of pancreatitis or inflammation of the pancreas.

Clofibrate: A medicine used to treat high triglycerides; also called Atromid®.

Clonidine: A medicine used to treat high blood pressure; also called Catapres®.

Clopidogrel: A blood thinner commonly prescribed for people after angioplasty or for people at risk for heart attack or stroke; also called Plavix®.

Clot: A clump of blood that has solidified as a result of a complex process involving platelets and various proteins; also called a *thrombus*, or *thrombosis*.

Colesevelam: A bile acid sequestrant used in the treatment of high cholesterol; also called WelChol®.

Colestipol: A bile acid sequestrant that is used to treat high blood levels of cholesterol; also called Colestid®.

Conduction system: The electrical system of the heart; the electric impulses that travel through the conduction system prompt the heart to contract and pump blood.

Coronary artery disease (CAD): Disease of the arteries supplying the heart muscle; usually involves blockages caused by the build-up of atherosclerotic plaque.

Defibrillation: The application of an electric shock to the heart to stop an abnormal heart rhythm.

Diastole: That portion of the heart cycle when the heart is relaxed.

Diastolic blood pressure: The pressure in the arteries while the heart is relaxed; it is the lower of the two numbers a doctor measures when taking blood pressure.

Digitalis: A medicine derived from the foxglove plant, used for centuries to treat heart failure.

Digoxin: A form of digitalis that is used to increase the pumping strength of the heart or to slow the pulse in atrial fibrillation; also called Lanoxin®.

Diltiazem: A medicine used to treat angina, high blood pressure, and certain abnormal heart rhythms; also called Cardizem®, Cartia®, Tiazac®, or Dilacor®.

Dipyridamole: A blood thinner; also called Persantine®.

Disopyramide: A medicine used to treat abnormal heart rhythms; also called Norpace® or Norpace CR®.

Diuretics: Medicines that increase urine output; they are used in the treatment of high blood pressure and heart failure.

Dofetilide: A medicine used to treat abnormal heart rhythms; also called Tikosyn®.

Doxazosin: A medicine used to treat high blood pressure; also called Cardura®.

Dyslipidemia: Abnormal levels of blood fats; also called *dyslipoproteinemia*.

Dyspnea: Shortness of breath.

Electrocardiogram (EKG): A graphic display of the electrical activity of the heart.

Electrophysiologic study (EPS): A special procedure performed in a laboratory in which catheters are inserted into the heart to test the heart's electrical system; sometimes an ablation of an abnormal focus of electrical activity is done during EPS.

Embolus (*pl.*emboli): A clot that has broken off and traveled from one place in the body to another; also called an *embolism*.

Enalapril: A medicine used to treat high blood pressure and heart failure; also called Vasotec®.

Endothelin: A naturally occurring substance that constricts arteries.

Epinephrine: A naturally occurring substance that is released in the body in response to stress; also called *adrenaline*.

Eplerenone: A diuretic used in the treatment of high blood pressure and congestive heart failure; also called Inspra®.

Eprosartan: An angiotensin receptor blocker (ARB) used to treat high blood pressure; also called Teveten®.

Ethacrynic acid: A diuretic used to treat high blood pressure and congestive heart failure; also called Edecrin®.

Ezetimibe: A medicine used to treat high cholesterol; also called Zetia®.

Fatty acids: Substances found in food that are used by the body to generate energy.

Felodipine: A calcium channel blocker (CCB) used to treat high blood pressure; also called Plendil®.

Fenofibrate: A medicine used to treat high triglycerides and high cholesterol; also called Tricor®.

Fibric acid derivatives: A class of medicines used to treat high blood lipids, particularly high triglycerides; also called *fibrates*.

Flecainide: A medicine used to treat abnormal heart rhythms; also called Tambocor®.

Fluvastatin: A medicine used to treat high blood cholesterol; also called Lescol®.

Fosinopril: An angiotensin converting enzyme (ACE) inhibitor used to treat high blood pressure; also called Monopril®.

Furosemide: A diuretic used to treat heart failure and high blood pressure; also called Lasix®.

Gemfibrozil: A medicine used to treat high blood levels of triglycerides; also called Lopid®.

Guanfacine: A medicine used to treat high blood pressure; also called Tenex®.

Heart failure: A condition in which the heart is unable to pump enough blood for the body's needs; can have many causes; also called *congestive heart failure*.

High-density lipoprotein (HDL): "Good" cholesterol; it helps protect against atherosclerosis.

Hydralazine: A medicine used to treat high blood pressure and congestive heart failure; also called Apresoline®.

Hydrochlorothiazide: A diuretic used to treat high blood pressure; also called Hydrodiuril®.

Hyperlipidemia: High levels of cholesterol and/or triglyceride; also called *hyperlipoproteinemia*.

Hypertension: High blood pressure.

Iloprost: A medicine used to treat primary pulmonary hypertension; also called Ventavis®.

Implantable cardiac defibrillator (ICD): *See* Automatic implantable cardiac defibrillator (AICD).

Indapamide: A diuretic used to treat high blood pressure; also called Lozol®.

Intermediate-density lipoprotein (IDL): A blood fat that is formed by the breakdown of very low-density lipoprotein.

Intima: The innermost layer of an artery; it is the first line of defense protecting the artery from harmful substances in the blood.

Irbesartan: An angiotensin receptor blocker (ARB) used to treat high blood pressure and congestive heart failure; also called Avapro®.

Ischemia: A condition in which the blood supply to an organ is not sufficient for the organ's needs.

Isosorbide: A medicine that dilates blood vessels; used in the treatment of angina and sometimes congestive heart failure; also called Isordil®, Sorbitrate®, Imdur®, Dilatrate-SR®, or Ismo®.

Isradipine: A calcium channel blocker used to treat high blood pressure; also called DynaCirc CR®.

Labetalol: A beta-blocker used to treat high blood pressure; also called Normodyne®, Trandate®.

Left ventricle: The pumping chamber on the left side of the heart.

Lipid: Another word for blood fats.

Lipoprotein: A blood fat joined to a protein.

Lisinopril: An ACE inhibitor used to treat high blood pressure and congestive heart failure; also called Zestril® or Prinivil®.

Losartan: An angiotensin receptor blocker (ARB) used to treat high blood pressure and heart failure; also called Cozaar®.

Lovastatin: The first "statin" medicine to be approved in the United States; used to treat high cholesterol; also called Mevacor®.

Low-density lipoprotein (LDL): The "bad" cholesterol; high levels increase the risk of atherosclerosis.

Lp(a): An altered blood fat that when elevated may be a risk factor for atherosclerosis.

Lumen: The passage in an artery or vein through which blood flows.

Methyldopa: An older blood pressure treatment rarely used today; also called Aldomet®.

Metolazone: A diuretic used to treat high blood pressure, and sometimes congestive heart failure; also called Zaroxolyn®.

Metoprolol: A beta-blocker used to treat angina, high blood pressure, heart failure, and certain abnormal heart rhythms; also called Toprol XL® or Lopressor®.

Minoxidil: A medicine used to treat high blood pressure; also called Loniten®.

Mitral valve: A one-way valve on the left side of the heart that is found between the left atrium and the left ventricle.

Moexipril: An ACE inhibitor used to treat high blood pressure; also called Univasc®.

Myalgia: Muscle pain; may be a side effect of statins.

Myocardial infarction (MI): Death of heart muscle due to interruption of its blood supply; usually caused by the rupture of a plaque with clot formation that totally blocks blood supply to a portion of the heart; also called a *heart attack.*

Myocardial ischemia: A condition in which the heart muscle is not getting enough blood supply for its needs; usually caused by blockages in the arteries supplying the heart.

Myocardium: A medical term for the heart muscle.

Nadolol: A beta-blocker medicine used to treat angina, high blood pressure, and certain abnormal heart rhythms; also called Corgard®.

Niacin: A B vitamin used to treat high triglycerides; also raises HDL cholesterol and lowers total and LDL cholesterol; also called nicotinic acid or Niaspan®.

Nicardipine: A calcium channel blocker used to treat high blood pressure; also called Cardene SR®.

Nicotine: A highly addictive chemical found in cigarettes and other forms of tobacco.

Nifedipine: A calcium channel blocker used to treat high blood pressure, angina, and pulmonary hypertension; also called Procardia® or Adalat®.

Nisoldipine: A calcium channel blocker used to treat high blood pressure; also called Sularl®.

Nitrates: A class of medicines that dilate blood vessels; used to treat angina.

Nitroglycerin: The most commonly prescribed nitrate used to treat angina.

Olmesartan: An angiotensin receptor blocker used to treat high blood pressure; also called Benicar®.

Omega-3 fatty acids: Compounds found in fish, canola oil, and walnuts. In high doses they lower triglycerides. The only prescription preparation of omega-3 fatty acids is called Omacor®.

Orthopnea: The occurrence of shortness of breath upon lying down; may be a symptom of congestive heart failure.

Oxygen: An element that is necessary for life; carried in the blood and given up by blood in the capillaries to nourish all the tissues of the body.

P wave: A part of the electrocardiogram that is caused by electricity traveling through the atria.

Pacemaker: A pacemaker is a structure that causes an electrical impulse to stimulate heart muscle. Natural pacemakers occur in the heart; if these fail, a doctor can insert an artificial pacemaker, which will stimulate the heart to beat.

Palpitations: A sensation of fluttering in the chest that is usually caused by extra heartbeats or abnormal heart rhythms.

Parasympathetic nervous system: A part of the nervous system that usually causes the heart rate to slow and the blood pressure to drop.

Penbutolol: A beta-blocker used to treat high blood pressure; also called Levatol®.

Perindopril: An angiotensin-converting enzyme (ACE) inhibitor used to treat high blood pressure; also called Aceon®.

Pindolol: A beta-blocker used to treat high blood pressure; also called Visken®.

Phosphodiesterase Type 5 (PDE 5) inhibitor: A group of medicines useful in the treatment of erectile dysfunction, one of which (sildenafil) has also been found to be effective in the treatment of primary pulmonary hypertension.

Plaque: A build-up of material composed of lipids, smooth muscle cells, and white blood cells in the walls of arteries, eventually causing the artery to be narrowed.

Platelets: Microscopic elements in the blood that are involved in the formation of clots.

Polythiazide: A diuretic used to treat high blood pressure; also called Renese®.

Potassium: A chemical element found in the blood and in cells; its levels are tightly regulated because levels that are either too high or too low can be dangerous.

Pravastatin: A statin medication used to treat high cholesterol; also called Pravachol®.

Prazosin: A medicine used to treat high blood pressure; also called Minipress®.

Premature contraction: A heartbeat coming sooner than normal; these can arise from the atria or the ventricles; also called a *premature beat.*

Primary pulmonary hypertension: *See* Pulmonary hypertension.

Procainamide: A medicine used to treat abnormal heart rhythms; also called Pronestyl® or Procan®.

Propafenone: A medicine used to treat abnormal heart rhythms; also called Rythmol® or Rythmol SR®.

Propranolol: A beta-blocker medicine used to treat angina and high blood pressure; also called Inderal® or Inderal LA®.

Prostacyclin: A prostaglandin that causes blood vessels to dilate.

Prostaglandins: A group of substances made by the body that have multiple effects on blood vessels, the inflammatory process, and blood clotting.

Pulmonary: A medical term for anything relating to the lungs.

Pulmonary artery: The artery that conducts venous blood from the right ventricle to the lungs.

Pulmonary hypertension (also called **Primary pulmonary hypertension**): A disease in which the pressure on the right side of the heart is elevated, eventually leading to heart failure.

Pulmonic valve: A one-way valve between the right ventricle and the pulmonary artery.

Pulse: The impulse that the contraction of the heart causes; it can be felt over various arteries, including those in the neck, wrist, groin, and feet.

Quinapril: An angiotensin-converting enzyme (ACE) inhibitor used to treat high blood pressure and congestive heart failure; also called Accupril®.

QRS complex: A deflection on the electrocardiogram caused by electricity traveling through the ventricles; also called a Q wave.

Radio-frequency ablation: The process of destroying abnormal tissue by applying radio waves that generate heat; usually done for abnormal heart rhythms.

Ramipril: An angiotensin-converting enzyme (ACE) inhibitor used to treat high blood pressure and congestive heart failure; also called Altace®.

Ranolazine: A medicine used to treat angina; also called Ranexa®.

Renin: An enzyme made by the kidney that is involved in the regulation of blood pressure.

Reserpine: An older blood pressure medicine, rarely used today; also called Serpalan.

Rhabdomyolysis: Severe muscle breakdown and damage; a rare but serious potential side effect of statins and fibrates.

Right ventricle: The pumping chamber on the right side of the heart.

Risk factor: Any characteristic that increases an individual's chance of developing a disease.

Rosuvastatin: A medicine used to treat high cholesterol; also called Crestor®.

Salicylates: Aspirin-like medicines.

Side effect: A symptom that may occur on taking a medication. Side effects can be trivial or very serious.

Sildenafil: A medicine used to treat pulmonary hypertension; also called Revatio®. (When used in a different dosage to treat erectile dysfunction, it is called Viagra®.)

Simvastatin: One of the statin medicines used to treat high cholesterol; also called Zocor®.

Sinus node: The normal pacemaker of the heart.

Sodium: A chemical element found in blood and cells that is regulated by the kidneys within narrow limits; levels that are too high or too low can be dangerous.

Sotalol: A medicine used to treat abnormal heart rhythms; also called Betapace® or Betapace AF®.

Spironolactone: A diuretic that is used in the treatment of high blood pressure and congestive heart failure; also called Aldactone®.

Statins: A class of medicines that is very effective in treating high cholesterol and decreasing the risk of heart attack, stroke, and cardiac death.

Sympathetic nervous system: The part of the nervous system involved in the "fight-or-flight" reflex; generally causes the pulse and blood pressure to rise.

Symptom: A feeling or manifestation that arises from a particular condition or disease. For example, itching can be a symptom of a rash.

Systole: The part of the heart's cycle in which the ventricles are contracting.

Tachycardia: An abnormally fast heart rate; also called a *tachyarrhythmia*.

Telmasartan: An angiotensin receptor blocker used in the treatment of high blood pressure; also called Micardis®.

Terazosin: A medicine used to treat high blood pressure; also called Hytrin®.

Thrombosis: The process of abnormal clot formation.

Thrombus (*pl.*thrombi): A clot occurring where it shouldn't be.

Ticlopidine: A blood thinner; also called Ticlid®.

Timolol: A beta-blocker used to treat angina and high blood pressure; also called Blockadren®.

Tocainide: A medicine used to treat abnormal heart rhythms; also called Tonocard®.

Torsemide: A diuretic used to treat high blood pressure and congestive heart failure; also called Demadex®.

Trandolapril: An angiotensin-converting enzyme (ACE) inhibitor used to treat high blood pressure and congestive heart failure; also called Mavik.

Trans fats: Artificial fats that raise levels of LDL cholesterol and lower levels of HDL cholesterol; also called *partially hydrogenated vegetable oils*.

Triamterene: A diuretic; also called Dyrenium®.

Tricuspid valve: The valve on the right side of the heart between the right atrium and the right ventricle.

Triglyceride: A blood fat; high levels increase the risk of atherosclerosis, particularly in women.

Valsartan: A medicine used to treat high blood pressure and congestive heart failure; also called Diovan®.

Valves: Structures in the heart that keep the blood flowing in the correct direction.

Varenicline: A medicine used to treat nicotine addiction; also called Chantix®.

Veins: Blood vessels that carry blood that has given up oxygen to the tissues and removed carbon dioxide from the tissues.

Ventricles: The pumping chambers in the heart; the right ventricle pumps blood to the lungs; the left ventricle pumps blood to the body.

Ventricular fibrillation: A rapidly fatal arrhythmia in which the heart quivers rather than contracts.

Ventricular tachycardia: An abnormally fast heart rhythm arising in the ventricle.

Verapamil: A calcium channel blocker used to treat angina, high blood pressure, and certain abnormal heart rhythms; also called Isoptin®, Calan®, or Covera®.

Very low-density lipoprotein (VLDL): A lipoprotein that is the main carrier of triglycerides in the blood.

Warfarin: A blood thinner, also called Coumadin®.

Afterword

In this book, I have attempted to give concise information about many of the medications that are used to prevent and treat cardiovascular disease. Like all medicines, those in this impressive armamentarium can both save and take lives. There has never been a medicine discovered or formulated that is totally free of risk. What your physician does when she or he prescribes a medicine is to weigh the possible risks versus the probable benefits. Only if the benefits outweigh the risks will she or he suggest that you start taking a drug. Ideally, you will have a discussion about the possible side effects, and the proper dosing schedule for your new medicine. You may be instructed to have blood tests to monitor the safety and efficacy of the drug. You will be told if any dietary changes need to be made to lessen the risk of side effects or to increase the benefit of the medicine. It is crucial that you have a good understanding of why the medicine has been prescribed and what you should do if you think you are having a side effect.

I insist that all of my patients carry an updated list of their medicines in their wallet. In fact, we provide a blank list at the first visit, then make a copy of it at each subsequent visit. This list gives the name of the medicine, the dosage, and the number of times a day the medicine needs to be taken. It should be shown to any doctor involved in your care so that he or she does not inadvertently prescribe a medicine that can cause an adverse interaction. I urge my patients not to stop taking any of their medicines without speaking to me first. Very often, what people think is a side effect is not; instead, it may be a symptom of the very condition I am treating them for.

After many years as a practicing physician, I have come to realize that a warm, trusting physician-patient relationship is every bit as important as medication. In my teaching rounds with doctors in training, I tell them that nothing they do for their patients is more important than listening—really listening, listening attentively, listening with their hearts as well as their minds, hearing not just the words that are said, but intuiting the fear, anxiety, and even anguish that is often present but not verbalized. Only by careful listening can the correct diagnosis be made. Only by careful listening can a physician understand not just the patient's illness but his or her human condition. When people believe that their physician cares for them, no matter what disease they are afflicted with, recovery is facilitated.

Your doctor cannot *make* you healthy but the two of you, working together, can maximize the likelihood that your acute problem will be alleviated and your chronic condition(s) will be controlled. Norman Cousins wrote: "Drugs are not always necessary. Belief in recovery always is. " If drugs *are* necessary, believing that your doctor cares what happens to you will make you more apt to take them as prescribed.

When illness supervenes or our bodies begin to fail as they inevitably must with advancing age, medicines can make possible years of useful, enjoyable life. I feel fortunate to practice in an era when so many effective drugs are available and I salute the many scientists and physicians who have provided these remedies to the suffering among us.

Index